THE NATURAL WAY SERIES

Increasing numbers of people worldwide are falling victim to illnesses which modern medicine, for all its technical advances, seems often powerless to prevent – and sometimes actually causes. To help with these so-called 'diseases of civilization' more and more people are turning to 'natural' medicine for an answer. The *Natural Way* series aims to offer clear, practical and reliable guidance to the safest, gentlest and most effective treatments available – and so to give sufferers and their families the information they need to make their own choices about the most suitable treatments.

Titles in the Natural Way *series*

Allergies
Arthritis & Rheumatism
Asthma
Back Pain
Cancer
Candida
Chronic Fatigue Syndrome
Colds & Flu
Cystitis
Diabetes
Eczema
Epilepsy
Hay Fever
Heart Disease
HIV and AIDS
Infertility
Irritable Bowel Syndrome
Migraine
Multiple Sclerosis
Premenstrual Syndrome
Psoriasis

THE NATURAL WAY

Psoriasis

Hilary Bower

Series medical consultants
Dr Peter Albright MD (USA)
& Dr David Peters MD (UK)

Approved by the
AMERICAN HOLISTIC MEDICAL ASSOCIATION
& BRITISH HOLISTIC MEDICAL ASSOCIATION

E L E M E N T
Shaftesbury, Dorset ● Boston, Massachusetts
Melbourne, Victoria

© Element Books Limited 1996
Text © Hilary Bower 1996

First published in the UK in 1996 by
Element Books Limited
Shaftesbury, Dorset SP7 8BP

Published in the USA in 1996 by
Element Books, Inc.
160 North Washington Street, Boston, MA 02114

Published in Australia in 1996 by
Element Books and distributed by
Penguin Australia Limited
487 Maroondah Highway,
Ringwood, Victoria 3134

Reissued 1998
Reprinted 1999

Cover Design by Slatter-Anderson
Designed and typeset by Linda Reed and Joss Nizan
Printed and bound in Great Britain

British Library Cataloguing in Publication data available

Library of Congress Cataloging in Publication
data available

ISBN 1 85230 832 X

Contents

List of illustrations   vi
Acknowledgements   viii
Introduction   ix

Chapter 1   **What is psoriasis?**   1
Chapter 2   **Different types of psoriasis**   10
Chapter 3   **What causes psoriasis?**   16
Chapter 4   **How to help yourself**   24
Chapter 5   **Conventional treatments and
             procedures**   37
Chapter 6   **The natural therapies
             and psoriasis**   47
Chapter 7   **Diet and environmental
             therapies**   56
Chapter 8   **Treating mind and emotions**   76
Chapter 9   **Therapies for healing the skin**   96
Chapter 10   **How to find and choose a
             practitioner**   116

Appendix A **Useful organizations**   125
Appendix B **Useful further reading**   130
Index   131

Illustrations

Figure 1	*The structure of the skin*	7
Figure 2	*Examples of UVB lamps suitable for home use*	33
Figure 3	*A Mora therapy unit*	51
Figure 4	*The three main autogenic positions*	85
Figure 5	*The meridian system in Chinese acupuncture*	104
Figure 6	*Acupressure points for psoriasis*	106
Figure 7	*Herbs for psoriasis*	110
Figure 8	*Reflex zones on the right foot*	114

Acknowledgements

Many people have helped in the writing of this book by talking freely of their knowledge and experiences. I would like to thank them all, including staff and members of the Psoriasis Association in Great Britain and Ireland; Judith Gay of 3J's Homoeopathy Clinic, London; Linda Lazarides of the Society for the Promotion of Nutritional Therapy; Dr Palle Rosted; and staff and therapists at the Hale Clinic, London and Cherryfields Clinic, Limerick (Eire).

Introduction

Psoriasis is a skin condition that has baffled doctors for many years. It can start at any time of life and shows up as anything from a few red spots on arms or legs to a covering of raw flaky skin all over the body. Naturally, this causes not only physical discomfort but also deep embarrassment, depression and shame for those who suffer the condition. Our skin is 'public property', and blemished skin can severely restrict our occupations, social activities, hobbies and relationships. Plus, psoriasis is a chronic condition, coming and going for no apparent reason, and sufferers are often left in an uncertain limbo, feeling unable to control their lives and doubting their self-worth and confidence.

There are many theories about what causes psoriasis – from complex genetics to diet and stress – but no one has yet pinned down exactly what triggers the disease. This makes it notoriously difficult to treat. Modern medicine is sometimes successful at relieving the symptoms, but it cannot offer a cure. Conventional therapy can mean years of unpleasant, smelly creams and potions, or of taking strong medicines which carry their own dangers for health. Some sufferers say it is hard to decide which is worse – the condition or the treatment.

But this need not be the end of the story. Natural medicine offers a whole new range of safe and effective options which have shown as good, and in some cases, better rates of success. Natural therapists use a 'holistic' approach that sees each individual as unique and takes into account everything about the patient, not just the skin symptoms. As a result many people have found relief in natural medicine after years of unsuccessful conventional treatments.

But natural medicine also requires you to take part. It is unlikely that therapy will involve just popping a pill or smoothing on a cream. You may be asked, with the help of your therapist, to change your daily routine, the food your eat, even the way you think. To do this you need to know that the person asking you to make these changes is trustworthy and has your well-being at heart.

Finding the right therapist and the right therapy can be bewildering – it can be hard to know where to find them, who is reliable and which treatments might suit you best. This book aims to be a guide to the sources of help available, discussing how they work, how effective they are, who provides them and what happens during consultations and treatments. And because you are the most important player in your health, it also offers suggestions for practical self-help.

Whichever therapy you try, remember two things. First, psoriasis is a very individual condition – a therapy that does not work on someone else may clear your skin completely; or if the first one doesn't work for you, try something else. Second, approaching the therapy of your choice with a positive attitude will not only give it much more chance of succeeding, but will benefit your health and you as a whole in many other ways.

CHAPTER 1

What is psoriasis?

How the skin works and why it goes wrong

Some people say the first thing they notice when meeting someone is the eyes. Others say it is the person's figure or voice. Almost all, however, underestimate the power of the skin to attract or repel.

As people with psoriasis know only too well, the skin is the major interface between us and the outside world. A clear, glowing, rosy skin draws people; they see it as a flag of health and well-being. But a blemished complexion seems to trigger all sorts of deep-seated fears of infection and illness. People can shy away from a handshake, from the adjacent seat on the bus – and even warn their children away. All this can be very distressing, particularly when you know that psoriasis is not an infection and is not contagious (catching).

So what is psoriasis? In physical terms, it is caused by an abnormality of the skin which increases both the speed at which skin cells are produced and the time they take to mature – that is, to reach the outside layers of the body (*see* page 8). This increased cell production is what causes the characteristic signs of psoriasis – dry, reddish patches covered with silvery scales which develop on any part of the body, but most often on the elbows, knees, scalp, nails and the lower back. Exactly why this speeding up takes place still puzzles many health professionals, but what is known, though, is that psoriasis is a *chronic* disorder. This means that once a person has a bout of it, they are likely to suffer future attacks, even though they may have long periods of clear skin.

Who gets psoriasis?

Between 2 and 3 per cent of the world's population have psoriasis – 80–120 million people. In the United States there are around 5–6 million psoriasis sufferers, in the UK 1.5 million, and in Australia around 500,000 cases. It appears to affect all races equally, with the exception of the native Indian populations of North and South America, and Greenland Eskimos (at least those who eat a diet based on cold-water fish; *see* page 22). Black-skinned peoples are also rarely affected when living in tropical climates, though they do suffer elsewhere.

Men and women are affected in the same proportion and are most likely to get psoriasis for the first time between the ages of 11 and 45.

The fact that well-known people are also affected by psoriasis shows that the condition needn't keep you out of the spotlight: British comedian Ben Elton, American writer John Updike, and Australian singer-actor Jason Donovan are all sufferers. (For Abimael Guzman, leader of the Peruvian terrorist group, The Shining Path, psoriasis caused more than skin-deep problems: he was captured during an incognito trip to a clinic in Lima.)

Psoriasis is no new disease. Medical archaeologists have found signs of typical psoriasis plaques on mummified bodies from 2,000 years ago. So, unlike many other skin conditions, psoriasis cannot be blamed on the increasing toxicity of chemicals in today's environment or specific elements of modern lifestyle, even though both may play a role.

What skin does

Skin is more than just a container for our insides. It keeps bugs, dust and water out, eliminates waste, filters the sun, balances the body's temperature, sends warning messages to the brain about the environment, provides a store of fat for warmth and food, and even creates the personal aroma that helps us attract our 'mate' – all within a thickness of about 5 millimetres (quarter of an inch).

It controls the moisture levels in our body, keeping harmful substances and moisture out, and the fluids and substances we need in. It allows us to let off steam – and all the toxic elements that build up day to day – through sweat.

Though skin is tough enough to withstand knocks, bumps, pricks and burns, it stays soft and pliable, even after constant washing. It renews its entire surface once a month. It can stretch to accommodate extra weight or a baby, then shrink back into shape. It repairs itself – notice how quickly cuts, scrapes, even surgical incisions heal – and even produces its own anti-bacterial and anti-fungal agents to prevent infection.

On top of all this, the skin is the largest organ in the body – weighing on average 4 kilograms (8 pounds 13 ounces) and covering an area of 2 square metres (2 square yards) – and is a major player in the 'cleaning systems' which filter and carry away the body's toxins and waste products.

For the skin to carry out this role properly, it has to function normally – and in psoriasis it does not. It is not known whether this malfunction is a *cause* of psoriasis or an *effect*. Complicating matters even further, the health of our skin is also affected by our mental health. Worry, grief, anxiety, stress and emotional strain all produce chemical reactions in the body which can take their toll on the skin. And, of course, psoriasis can cause all these emotions too. In this way the condition can be seen as a vicious circle (*see* page 80).

Function of the skin

- puts a protective barrier between the environment and the body
- keeps body temperature constant
- eliminates waste minerals, fluids and toxins
- prevents dehydration
- gives early warning of attack to the immune system
- reports sensations to the brain

The structure of skin

What you see in the mirror and call your skin is actually several layers of old, dead cells (the building blocks of the body) that have interlocked to form a protective layer for the living system below – rather like a tile roof over a house. Underneath that 'roof' are two layers of skin, each of which plays a different role in the health of your body (*see* fig.1).

The epidermis

The top layer of skin – the one you see in the mirror – is called the *epidermis*. Although it may not look or feel like it, this layer is extremely tough. It is made largely of *keratin*, a hard-wearing protein which is made by cells as they move up through the layers of skin. Keratin also forms nails and hair, but in the skin it is kept supple by the secretions of various glands which have outlet points in the epidermis.

Once these cells reach the surface they create the horny coat which protects the sensitive layers below against damage, disease, chemicals and other potential dangers. This 'roof' also prevents dehydration, and without it we would be dead in a few hours. But the cells are also dead and dry and fall off continuously, creating most of what we know as household dust. As they fall off they are replaced by cells from below, which means that about once a month you have an entirely new skin.

The epidermis also houses *melanocytes*; these cells are responsible for producing a substance in the skin called *melanin*, which helps protect against the sun's harmful rays. When the skin is exposed to the sun, melanocytes produce more melanin and, if you give your skin cells time to swing into operation, they inject surrounding cells with enough melanin to provide a degree of natural sunscreen. But if you expose your skin to the sun too rapidly, these specialized cells have no time to increase their production and the skin gets sunburnt.

Other special cells in the epidermis are *Langerhans cells*, which give the immune system early warning of an attack by, for instance – viruses or airborne *allergens* (substances that cause allergies), and *Merkel cells*, which help the brain to recognize sensations of touch and feeling.

The dermis

The middle layer of the skin, the *dermis*, is where the real work of the skin is carried out. This layer is the web of elastic fibres, blood vessels, hair roots and follicles, nerve endings, sweat and lymph glands, that allows the skin to do its job of getting rid of all the poisons and toxins the body creates during the process of ordinary day-to-day living. The thickness of the dermis depends on where it is and what other elements it contains. It is thickest on the palms of the hands and the soles of the feet, and thinnest in the eyelids.

The tissue in the dermis is made of *collagen* and *elastin*. Not only do these substances form the web that holds all the other elements, they also determine how youthful – or otherwise – your skin looks. They provide the skin with its strength and stretchiness and allow it to accommodate changing weight and size. But the ability of these substances to return to shape diminishes with age, which is why those dreaded wrinkles and sags start to appear. Some researchers say how we age depends on our genetic programming, but there is also evidence that factors such as smoking and pollution, an unhealthy diet and too much sunbathing, can also make the skin age before its time.

Dotted throughout the dermis are the *eccrine* or sweat glands, which produce about half a litre of sweat a day; and *lymph* glands, which drain away excess proteins. Sweat has two roles: it carries out waste, salts and toxins through tiny openings (pores) in the epidermis; and it cools the skin as it evaporates on the surface, thus playing a vital role in the body's temperature balance. Eccrine glands increase their output as much as ten times during exercise or in hot weather.

The skin's blood supply also runs through this layer. In hot conditions, the tiny blood vessels (*capillaries*) which loop through the dermis expand to increase the flow and bring warm blood from the body's core to the surface to cool. In cold weather the opposite happens – the capillaries contract to keep as much warmth as possible in the body.

Hair follicles are another occupant of the dermis, and along with these are the *sebaceous* glands, which produce greasy *sebum* to lubricate and waterproof the skin. Sebum also has mild anti-bacterial and anti-fungal properties. *Apocrine* glands are a type of sweat gland found in the hair follicles of the breasts, armpits and groin. They are usually activated around puberty and produce the special individualized odour that many people believe is the root of sexual attraction. However, it can also become unpleasantly smelly if left to go stale on the skin.

Lastly, the dermis houses a huge number of nerve endings which help the brain to interpret what's going on around us and to identify sensations such as heat, cold, rough, smooth, pressure, pain and itching.

Underneath all this is a layer of fatty tissue which is basically a body 'cushion', protecting our internal organs from bumps and knocks, insulating us from heat and cold, and providing a store house of fat which we can call on in bad times.

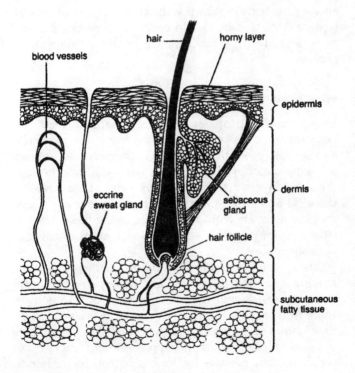

Fig. 1 The structure of the skin

The life-cycle of a skin cell

Like all body tissues, the skin's two layers are made up of hundreds of thousands of cells. New cells are continuously created in the deepest layer of the skin, and over three to four weeks they are pushed up through the dermis and the epidermis, maturing as they go, until they finally reach the surface. After spending a while as part of the 'roof' layer of the epidermis, the dead cells are shed as scales and new ones take their place. This process of renewal is constant and normally well balanced – the body creates just the right number of cells to replace those that are lost. In people with psoriasis, however, something goes haywire in this replacement process.

What happens to psoriasis cells?

In people with psoriasis two things happen. First, the body for some reason generates too many new skin cells and second, psoriatic cells live a high-speed life. Instead of taking a month to mature, the new cells race through the skin's layers in five to six days – so fast that they are still alive and kicking when they reach the surface. There they amalgamate with dead cells, causing the characteristic signs of psoriasis – raw, red skin patches covered with silver scales.

These patches change the nature of the epidermis, making it not only thicker but also more permeable, both from the inside and the outside. The body thus loses more fluid, which can escape through psoriatic skin up to ten times faster than through normal skin. This causes the skin to lose much of its suppleness, and cracks occur where the skin needs to be flexible, such as on the hands, feet and elbows. At the same time these changes give bacteria and other 'invaders' a better chance of penetrating the body, causing other skin problems.

Because more cells are being produced, more cells are dying and falling off as scales than usual. One man who finally found a successful alternative treatment for his psoriasis said his greatest joy was being able to stay in other people's houses or in hotels without leaving bushels of embarrassing scabs everywhere, and being able to take his shirt off in hot weather without frightening the neighbours!

Changes also take place in the dermis. In psoriasis the capillaries widen, making the blood-flow to the skin much greater than normal. This is why psoriasis patches are red and bleed particularly easily. The blood also contains an unusually high number of white cells – the 'fighter' cells produced by the immune system to protect the body when it is attacked by viruses, infections or allergens. The increased amount of white cells adds to the inflammatory process, although it is not the cause of it.

What causes the skin to overreact in this way has so far confounded many experts. But there are plenty of theories, some of which are discussed in chapter 3.

CHAPTER 2

Different types of psoriasis

What they look like and who gets them

There are many different forms of psoriasis. It can appear anywhere on the body – legs, arms, back, scalp, even the nails – though it is, thankfully, quite rare on the face.

Some people have different types of psoriasis at different times in their life; some have the odd patch, often in one consistent place, which comes and goes; others find larger areas of the body are troubled. In the worst cases, the whole body can be affected with serious eruptions and hospital care may be necessary.

Psoriasis is what's called a 'chronic' condition: it is likely to come and go for unpredictable periods over a person's lifetime. About a third of people with psoriasis are naturally clear of the condition for long periods of time and only need treatment when it recurs. Sometimes there is an obvious reason for these recurrences – perhaps an injury to the skin or a period of intense anxiety (*see* trigger factors in Chapter 3). At other times it can seem like the skin has a mind of its own, flaring up angrily or clearing miraculously for no apparent reason.

In fact, the occasions when the skin seems to be reacting to some invisible prompt can be a useful time for psoriasis sufferers to take a close look at what is happening in their lives and their environment to see if they can pick up clues as to what might be behind their condition (the skin often mirrors psychological or physical problems that are otherwise hidden). A flare-up may be a tip-off to a food allergy or to a stress reaction that they have become so used to that they are not aware of it any more, although it is still wreaking havoc on their well-being (*see* pages 59 and 79).

Psoriasis can sometimes be confused with eczema. In this condition the skin becomes inflamed after contact with a harsh or irritating substance, or because of an allergy, or both. Though it can have similar effects on the skin, eczema is quite a different condition and is more easily treated once the cause of the inflammation has been identified. More information on this condition can be found in *The Natural Way: Eczema*.

Plaque (or discoid) psoriasis

Plaque psoriasis is the most common type – around 90 per cent of psoriasis sufferers have this form. The skin develops clearly defined patches of pink or red skin called *plaques*, which are covered with dry, crusty, silvery scales which flake off.

Because the plaques are formed from cells that have come to the surface too quickly, they may be sticky as well as flaky, and scraping the scales off can make the skin bleed. Also, the presence of these live cells means there is increased blood-flow to the skin's surface, which can reduce body temperature, particularly if there are a lot of lesions. As a result, people with widespread plaques need to use a lot of energy to maintain their warmth and can consequently feel quite exhausted.

Plaque psoriasis most commonly occurs on the elbows, knees, lower back and scalp – and one side of the body often mirrors the other. However, it can show up anywhere, particularly if the skin has been bruised or injured.

The scalp is a common site and can be particularly difficult to deal with because of the irritation caused by washing the hair and the difficulty of applying soothing creams in this area. It does not usually affect hair growth.

Guttate psoriasis

This type of psoriasis is usually seen in children and teenagers and can be the first sign of a susceptibility to the condition. The name comes from the Latin word *gutta*, meaning drop, and the skin often looks like it has been splattered with drops of red paint from a brush.

In a flare-up numerous small round red spots appear suddenly, usually on the body rather than the limbs and scalp, and often a week or so after a sore throat or tonsillitis.

Though it can look dire, guttate psoriasis is one of the easiest patterns of psoriasis to treat if caught promptly. A little coal tar lotion or cream, together with coal tar bath oil and either sunshine or a short course of ultraviolet light, will usually do the trick.

If left untreated, however, guttate psoriasis can develop into plaque psoriasis. And even when treated, one in four children who have had guttate psoriasis will have further episodes of psoriasis in later life.

Flexural psoriasis

Flexural psoriasis is found in the folds of the body, such as under the breasts, between the buttocks, in the groin and where the legs and arms bend. The patches are inflamed and red like those in plaque psoriasis, but because of friction at the site, they are not usually scaly.

This type of psoriasis tends to occur more in older people, particularly women. It can, however, have knock-on effects. One man with severe psoriasis around the groin, for example, had difficulty fathering a child. Eventually he was found to have a low sperm-count, which doctors put down to the heat generated by the plaques around his scrotum. When the plaques cleared, in this case by using a special diet (*see* page 57 and 62), his other problem was also solved.

'Napkin' psoriasis

There is some debate whether this is in fact psoriasis at all. As the name suggests, it usually occurs in the nappy or diaper area in infants. It can also spread to other parts of the child's body, particularly to the scalp or moist folds of skin such as those under the arms. Some doctors believe babies who suffer from this condition have an increased risk of psoriasis later in life, but research evidence has not shown a clear link.

Nail psoriasis

Nail psoriasis is more common in people over 40. It is a good predictor of who will develop psoriatic arthritis (see below) as 80 per cent of people with nail psoriasis also develop joint inflammation.

This form of psoriasis arises when overactive cells produce a build-up of keratin, the substance that helps build and protect nails and hair. Nails generally become pitted like a thimble, or ridged, and they may also start to lift away from the finger, thicken and discolour.

Localized pustular psoriasis

More common in adults than in children, this type of psoriasis shows up as pus-filled spots, generally on the palms and soles. It is a cross-over with eczema, and is sometimes described as 'vesicular dermatitis', 'dyshidrotic eczema' or, more commonly, 'pompholyx'. The spots start off white and turn yellow, then brown. They are often painful and resist treatment. Sudden withdrawal from steroid therapy can cause this condition, and it is also linked to stress and fungal infections such as 'athlete's foot'. In severe cases patients may need to be admitted to hospital for a period of time.

Erythrodermic psoriasis

This is a serious, even life-threatening condition, though a rare one. Large areas of the skin become inflamed and scaly and patients lose the ability to control their body temperature and fluid loss. They become dehydrated and feverish and have an increased risk of infection and heart and kidney failure. Hospital care is vital.

Psoriatic arthritis

Around 6 per cent of people with psoriasis develop psoriatic arthritis, a condition in which the joints become stiff, painful and inflamed. It differs from other forms of arthritis in the pattern of joints that are affected. With psoriatic arthritis, an entire finger or toe typically becomes swollen, rather than an individual joint, but usually only one set of joints is affected. Common sites are the hands (particularly the very end joints of the fingers), feet, spine and neck. Bone destruction also tends to occur earlier in psoriatic arthritis than in other forms of arthritis.

The more severe the psoriasis, the more likely the subsequent development of arthritis. People with nail psoriasis are particularly likely to develop it, usually in the same fingers. In other cases, however, there seems to be no relationship between the site of the psoriasis on the skin and the joint which becomes inflamed.

As with the skin condition, psoriatic arthritis is a chronic condition which comes and goes. Sometimes the arthritis may flare up when the psoriasis itself is clear. Sometimes the tendons in an area become inflamed (*tendonitis*) with no sign of joint inflammation (*arthritis*).

Both sexes are equally affected, but men seem to be more prone to spinal arthritis. Women psoriasis sufferers may find that hormonal changes experienced during pregnancy or the menopause can trigger arthritis.

CHAPTER 3

What causes psoriasis?

Investigating the puzzle

The simple answer to what causes psoriasis is that no one knows for sure. There are plenty of theories – some based on pure science, some on environmental factors, others on psychological insights – but no certainties. What is certain is that problems with skin are rarely related just to something that is happening to the skin. The condition of the skin is intimately linked to what goes on in the rest of the body and the mind. In the end there will probably be elements of truth in all the theories – it is unlikely that such a complex condition as psoriasis has only one cause.

All in the genes?

Around 40 per cent of people with psoriasis have relatives who also suffer from the condition to some extent. So it is clear that something in the pattern of genes must play a role in causing psoriasis.

A child who has one parent with psoriasis has a 25 per cent chance of developing the same condition. This increases to 60 per cent if both parents are affected. If a child whose parents are not affected develops psoriasis, there is a 20 per cent chance that other children in the family will also develop the disease. The fact that some people do not develop psoriasis until later in life does not rule out a genetic cause – many inherited disorders stay hidden for a number of years.

Some geneticists believe that the answer may lie with a fault on one particular gene which affects the rate of cell production. Others believe a combination of several gene abnormalities may be needed to produce psoriasis. As for those people who have no afflicted family members and whose psoriasis seems to come out of the blue, scientists speculate that they could have been born with a new mutation or pattern of genes caused by a mistake in the gene set-up, or that maybe there are genes that only function abnormally in certain circumstances. But research has yet to prove any of these theories.

The immune system

The immune system is the body's defence mechanism. It has to recognize which substances are part of the body (self) and which are not (non-self), so that when it comes into contact with something it does not recognize as self (such as a bacteria, a splinter or a new heart), it can reject it. This is why people receiving an organ transplant have to take potent drugs to block the immune system, sometimes for the rest of their lives. The symptoms of a cold – a runny nose and a temperature – tell us that our body is fighting the virus. Sometimes, however, for reasons not yet fully understood, the immune system gets muddled and starts rejecting some of the body's own constituents. This results in *auto-immune* disorders.

Some scientists believe psoriasis is an auto-immune disorder because they have found far more of the chemicals that are circulated by the immune system when it is under attack in the skin of people with psoriasis than in normal skin. These chemicals are circulated via the plentiful nerve endings in the skin. They have also found more *t-helper cells* – a type of white blood cell which sends messages to the immune system when something is threatening the body.

As a test to see if this theory made any sense, Dr Eugene Farber from the Psoriasis Research Institute in Palo Alto, California, kept track of a patient who had psoriasis on both knees. The lesions on one knee disappeared after surgery temporarily damaged the nerve endings, leaving them unable to circulate the immune system chemicals. This knee was also left numb. Eighteen months later the sensation in the knee came back, but so did the plaques, showing that, in this case at least, the nerve endings had some connection with the man's psoriasis.

So, one theory says that the immune system itself is faulty in a person with psoriasis, because it reacts in the wrong way to substances which it should recognize as 'self'. Another theory, however, suggests that in psoriasis the body produces too much of a particular substance and the immune system sees this as a threat to the body's health.

Drug therapies that inhibit the immune system tend to be effective in clearing up psoriasis, but they also tend to have unpleasant side-effects. However, there are other ways to influence the immune system, both positively and negatively. Emotional states such as anger, grief, exhaustion, depression and anxiety can change the way it responds. For example, Dr Farber found stressful life-events increased the amount of *neuropeptides* (another immune chemical) in the brain, blood and skin. Luckily the reverse also seems to be true and positive attitudes, relaxation and pleasure can calm the body and help it find balance again (*see* Chapter 8).

Liver overload

Many complementary therapists, particularly those who deal with diet and food-related problems, believe that liver overload is a key factor in psoriasis. Researchers at

King's College Hospital, London, also found that a high percentage of psoriasis sufferers had a weakness in the liver.

The poisons and toxins which are created after food has been digested are carried through the body in the bloodstream. The liver picks them out and sends them on to be processed and disposed of through the 'waste disposal' systems – the bowel and bladder. But if the liver is overloaded or weakened, perhaps due to mineral deficiencies, over-indulgence in fatty foods or alcohol, or past injury, the toxins stay in the blood and recirculate. It is then possible that the skin, another of the body's waste disposal systems, tries to rid the body of its toxin overload and also becomes overworked, causing the skin reactions seen in psoriasis.

The build-up of toxins that weakens the liver can be caused by the food we eat, the air we breath, the water we drink, medication, stress levels, and so on (*see* page 60 for various methods of detoxifying the body).

The food we eat

Liver overload is not the only dietary explanation. Some natural therapists say that a diet high in meat, dairy products, sugar, processed foods, alcohol, and stimulants like caffeine, causes bad digestion, increases toxins and does not provide enough nutrients. When the body is running on empty, so too are the immune and central nervous systems, they argue.

It has also been suggested that psoriasis may be caused if proteins are not digested properly. When proteins do not break down, bacteria in the intestines produce a whole army of toxic compounds (*polyamines*) to fight them. These compounds play a role in sparking-off excessive cell division, which is what happens in psoriatic skin.

Some therapists specifically blame high consumption of animal fats in meat and dairy products for psoriasis. Studies have found that the skin of psoriasis sufferers contains high levels of compounds called *leucotrienes*, which cause inflammation. These are created by the body from *arachidonic* acid, which is found exclusively in animal fats. In some studies *eicosapentaenoic* acid (EPA), which is found in fish oils (*see* page 62), has been shown to slow down the production of leucotrienes. This is why some therapists promote EPA as a treatment. Other therapists believe that individual food allergies are a root cause because of how they affect the immune system. Chapter 7 discusses foods and their effect on psoriasis in more detail.

Mind power

It is thought that stress is the trigger factor for over 50 per cent of psoriasis sufferers. A number of carefully conducted studies have found that large numbers of people develop psoriasis for the first time after some stressful event or period in their lives, and that flare-ups are closely linked to stressful times. There are many different causes of stress:

- *Physical* – illness, an accident, an operation, exhaustion, a chronic disease such as psoriasis or asthma
- *Mental* – work, school, overtime, responsibility, finances, lack of confidence
- *Emotional* – relationships, marital problems, family disagreements, death of someone close, illness

Some people develop psoriasis at the time of their first major school examination, at the death of a close relative, or after taking on a new and challenging job. Others get flare-ups after arguments, work meetings, or when their bank balance goes into the red.

But this doesn't mean it is 'all in the mind'. Dr Farber in California found stressful events increased the amounts of immune system chemicals in the brain, blood and skin; and other scientists have found there is a marked difference in electrical brain patterns, blood pressure, pulse rates, hormone levels, and heart and intestinal activity when people are under stress. Plus, when we are not feeling happy we don't eat properly, we drink and smoke, we don't exercise, we dwell on our problems, and so on. All these things reduce the efficiency of all our biological systems and make us tired and irritable and less able to cope – in other words, more stressed. It's a vicious circle.

But if the mind is able to have such a strong negative influence, it stands to reason that it can have also the reverse effect. *See* Chapter 8 for how your mind and emotions can help to heal your skin.

Drawbacks of a sophisticated life

Some people believe that the Western lifestyle is a cause of psoriasis. Not only do we put pressure on our body systems with processed foods, alcohol, smoking and high-pressure lives, they say, but the chemical environment we live in is very different from the surroundings our bodies were fine-tuned to survive in. While food allergies have been recognized for years, many more people are now becoming sensitive to chemicals in the environment.

Proponents of this theory point to lead in water pipes and car exhausts, pesticides and industrial pollution that contaminate crops and air, food additives, potent fumes from household cleaners, dry cleaning fluids, photocopy machines, 'electromagnetic' pollution from power cables, microwaves and computers – all of which our immune system has to fight. And while in many cases our bodies are able to combat this onslaught effectively, for those whose immune system is weakened, perhaps by a virus or stress, there comes a time when it collapses and diseases such as psoriasis start to occur.

There is some evidence that those who live more simple lifestyles are less susceptible to psoriasis. Research on 26,000 South American Indians in 95 villages throughout Bolivia, Peru, Ecuador and Venezuela, found not one single case of psoriasis. Australian Aborigines had no record of psoriasis until they moved into Western society, and the condition is rare in Greenland Eskimos (although this may be because they eat a lot of cold-water fish which contains high levels of EPA).

Trigger factors

Whichever causal theory you subscribe to, it seems that psoriasis needs a 'trigger' to set it off in the first place and to provoke its unpredictable recurrences. Almost everyone has a different opinion as to what these trigger factors might be – and any combination of the following may be to blame.

● *Throat infections* – one of the two commonly identified triggers for psoriasis. This may be because these infections (such as tonsillitis, caused by the *streptococcus* bacteria) place a great burden on the immune system. In the UK, studies in Manchester found that two out of every five children who developed guttate psoriasis had had a recent streptococcal infection. One in four children who get guttate psoriasis go on to develop plaque psoriasis, though most will not be severely affected. Prompt treatment of sore throats with an antibiotic may stop the condition developing or help to reduce the severity of the flare-up.

- *Stress* – the other most common trigger. Stressful life-events (weddings, funerals, exams, arguments, new jobs, redundancy) have all been related to a first flare-up and to subsequent episodes.
- *Physical hurt* – violent scratching, flesh injuries, or wounds from surgical operations.
- *Hormones* – fluctuating hormone levels that accompany pregnancy, the menopause, or going on the contraceptive pill.
- *Alcohol* – possibly the final straw for a weakened liver.
- *Drugs* – anti-malarials, lithium and beta-blockers, for example. Systemic steroids or strong topical steroids may also trigger psoriasis, not only when they are taken but also when they are suddenly stopped.
- *Sunlight* – usually beneficial, but can cause a flare-up in about 10 per cent of psoriasis sufferers.

CHAPTER 4

How to help yourself

Living with psoriasis

Psoriasis – even small patches – can make you feel pretty bad. We're all bombarded with images of the body beautiful and its flawless skin, and though *you* know psoriasis is not contagious and that you haven't got it because you are dirty or sick in some way, short of wearing a sandwich board and handing out leaflets, you can feel that you'll never get other people to understand.

Some people feel they have lost control of their lives – they don't go swimming because of the way people look at them, they hate the supermarket because the assistant takes the money from their hand with distaste, and they have to spend embarrassing minutes explaining to the hairdresser that 'it's not catching'. Some people lose confidence, get down and depressed – guaranteed not to improve their skin – and begin to depend on what the doctor doles out to them.

But there are day-to-day things you can do for your skin to get that control back and approach life more positively.

Being a detective

With skin complaints, there is often a sense of the skin being 'rubbed up the wrong way' by the environment. But while the picture the body paints on its surface may not be welcome or pretty, it can be useful in tracking down something that disagrees with you.

It could be something physical like a perfume or a hand lotion, a food or additive, certain plants, or 'something in the air' such as pollen or pollution. But, particularly with psoriasis, it could also be a mental state. Your lesions may get worse after an argument, if you are under a lot of pressure, or when you are anxious, tired or embarrassed. Some people react badly when they are in a situation where they have no control over what happens next; others are the opposite – their skin flares up if they have to take responsibility.

By finding out what physical substances your skin reacts to, you can avoid those things. It is not quite as easy to avoid situations or feelings, but if you know what it is that winds you up, you can start looking for strategies to lessen the stress. For example, if your lesions flare up every time you feel nervous or unsure, you may want to seek out ways of improving your confidence and to help you take things in your stride (*see* below and Chapter 8).

Stress-busters

Stress, as discussed in Chapter 3, is a key trigger factor in psoriasis. This means psoriasis sufferers are often in a vicious circle – stressful situations trigger a flare-up, and flare-ups make for a stressful life. In addition to the stress of psoriasis there are all the normal things we worry about – mortgages and money and children and careers. Developing some stress-busting activities can help break the cycle, and if your skin starts to improve, your state of mind and ability to cope with other aspects of life are likely to improve too.

'Stress-busters' are quite individual – some people wind down by running, some by reading, some do incredibly complex crosswords or embroidery. You could meditate or use 'affirmations' (*see* Chapter 8 for how these work), or you could just put your feet up and daydream. In essence, take a little time each day to relax.

You'll also need some strategies for dealing with the high-stress situations that crop up without warning. It's important to be able to recognize when you are getting stressed, and to have some conscious actions that you can take to block that feeling. This could be anything from taking five slow, deep breaths to giving yourself a few minutes to stretch and relax your body.

Strategies to beat stress

- *Make lists* Lists avert panic and stop you worrying that you'll forget something important.
- *Plan ahead* Anticipate pressurized situations and look for solutions before you get to them.
- *Don't over commit yourself* No one can do everything – prioritize if you have a lot to do.
- *Spend some time outside every day* A quick walk around the block is better than nothing.
- *Look around you* Enjoy for a few seconds something that reminds you of the rest of the world – blue sky, trees changing colour, flowers blossoming, children playing, music.
- *Talk to a good friend* If you are worried about something, share your emotions rather than bottling them up. If you don't feel comfortable doing this, write them down.

Taking care of your skin

Any substance that comes into contact with your skin has the potential to either help or hurt it. So, as soon as you notice your skin is reacting differently – perhaps the flaking increases or the lesions redden, itch or even bleed – become a detective and try to track down which of the substances you have been in contact with could be responsible.

For example, some washing powders are quite abrasive, particularly if they contain 'biological' enzymes. The same goes for fabric conditioners, though we are persuaded to believe they are soft and gentle. And remember, you come into contact with any harmful ingredients not only when you're hand washing but also when you wear the clothes. If you are sensitive to one brand, try another, perhaps one made for sensitive skins.

The same applies to detergents, soaps, deodorants, shampoos, cosmetics, shaving foams, and so on. It is a good idea to start reading product labels – you may be able to identify particular additives that cause you trouble and thus avoid them from the beginning. Lanolin, for example, is a common ingredient in cosmetics and one that many people are allergic to. On the other hand, you may also identify certain things that help. Some psoriasis sufferers, for example, find soaps containing extract of aloe vera are soothing.

Generally speaking, it is better to seek out 'natural' brands since they generally contain fewer additives and perfumes. Natural medicine clinics often stock these product lines. But remember, products that claim to be for sensitive skins may still contain things your skin doesn't like. Don't rule them out in your detective work just because they are natural.

Moisturizers and bath oils

While you need to avoid harmful products, it is also important to find some that will help nurture and protect your skin. Soothing moisturizing creams (*emollients*) help prevent dryness – not by adding fluid but by preventing what is there escaping. They may help control scaling, though they do not have any effect on the underlying disease process. It is best to use simple non-scented products (*see* box).

Over-the-counter products

Sufferers have found the following products particularly useful: Pharbifarm (Sweden, also available in UK), Millcreek (US), and Marks and Spencer's Extracts of Nature (UK). Pharmaceutical manufacturers such as Dermal Laboratories (Emulsiderm) and Goldshield (Imuderm) have ranges of mild treatment ointments, lotions and bathroom preparations. All these products are available in most good pharmacies. In addition, there are:

Soap substitutes
- Crookes Wash E45 – contains zinc oxide and mineral oils
- Aqueous cream BP (also an emollient) and emulsifying ointment BP

Bath products
- Bath E45 and Savlon Bath Oil – unperfumed bath oils based on mineral oils
- Oilatum emollient and gel – liquid paraffin base
- Balneum – soya oil base
- Pixol solution – coal tar and cade oil (can be used in baths, showers or as scalp treatment)

Emollients and barrier creams
- Aqueous cream BP
- Herbamin – vaseline, liquid paraffin and essential minerals
- Cream E45 – petroleum jelly, liquid paraffin, lanolin
- Oilatum cream – arachis oil base
- Unguentum Merck – contains petroleum jelly (also for use before bathing)
- Hydromol – cream and emollient bath additive containing liquid paraffin, sodium ingredients and arachis oil

Shampoos
- Alphosyl – coal tar and alcohol extract
- Denorex – coal tar and menthol
- Ceanel concentrate – cetrimide, undecenoic acid and phenylethyl alcohol shampoo (can also be used on other parts of the body)

Over-the-counter treatments

- Potter's Psorasolv – traditional herbal ointment containing sulphur, zinc oxide, poke root extract and clivers soft extract
- Potter's skin eruptions mixture – herbal medicine for symptom relief containing extracts of cascara, blue flag, burdock root, yellow dock, sarsaparilla and buchu
- Psorin ointment and scalp gel – salicylic acid, dithranol and coal tar
- Gelcosal – salicylic acid, coal tar and pine tar (may help reduce heavy scaling)
- Polytar and Gelcotar liquids (for scalp plaques)

It is also a good idea to apply an emollient oil before a bath or shower, because although hot water can make you feel good, the harsh elements (particularly in city water) can be very drying. Or you can add an oil to the bath water. Some have ingredients that prevent or relieve itching (*antipuritics*).

Essential oils – distilled from the roots, leaves or flowers of plants and used in aromatherapy – can also be combined with bath oils. Lavender is thought to help restore the skin. It has also been shown to stimulate the brain's 'alpha' rhythms, the type of brain wave-pattern that occurs during relaxation. Remember, though, essential oils are not perfumes but complex chemical substances. Six to eight drops of neat oil are enough for a whole bath, and it's a good idea to mix it with a bath oil so that your skin is moisturized as well. (*See* page 75 for other natural bath additives that help.)

It is also possible to buy packs of natural mineral salts or muds, such as those from the Dead Sea, which may soothe the skin. One product, Mamina, comes from an Andean spring and has been used successfully in a leading hospital in Chile to treat skin disorders. It contains a blend of magnesium, calcium, potassium, sodium, nitrogen, sulphur, phosphorus, boron and zinc soluble salts. Normal bubble baths are not a good idea – they usually contain lots of detergent.

Hands and feet

It is best to wear gloves for gardening, household chores, home improvements, and so on. Avoid water that is too hot, even with gloves on, and always wear cotton gloves inside rubber gloves to prevent perspiration causing irritation. For the same reason, wear cotton socks inside shoes or boots, especially rubber boots. Ideally, wear leather footwear to allow your feet to breathe. Use plenty of moisturizer and a barrier cream to keep flaking to a minimum, and marigold oil if you have psoriasis of the nails – this is a healing remedy as well.

Scalp

Psoriasis tends to be more itchy on the scalp than anywhere else, and ordinary shampoos can irritate the already sensitive skin. Many psoriasis sufferers try dandruff shampoos, but not only can these be particularly harsh, they do little to reduce the flaking and can make it worse by drying out the scalp. Look for shampoos that use natural foaming substances, such as marshmallow flower, rather than detergents and conditioners based on natural moisturizers like henna wax.

Home-made herbal rinses may soothe both itching and flaking on the scalp without damaging the hair or making it look greasy and unattractive. Try soaking chickweed, marigold and nettle plants in warm water, then strain and use the cooled liquid to rinse. Or mix 10 millilitres of rosemary tincture and ten drops of cade oil in 500 millilitres of warm water for a final rinse.

Some practitioners say people in families susceptible

to psoriasis should try not to stress their scalp. This means avoiding hair dyes and perms, vigorous brushing or using tight curlers. But if you take your own shampoo and conditioner along to an understanding hairdresser, you may be able to enjoy the experience without too many repercussions. Hairdressers may also be able to help you find gentle perms and dye products, so that you don't have to miss out on hair experiments altogether.

Fabrics

Once again the best choice is a natural one. Materials such as cotton, wool and silk allow the skin to breathe and help prevent irritation. Synthetic fibres cause sweating which can increase flaking. Natural fibres are particularly important when choosing underwear and bed linen. For those with scalp psoriasis it can be a good idea to wear a light scarf because it can be shaken easily. Troubles with metals in jewellery and watches can be avoided by painting the surface that touches the skin with a hypo-allergenic paint. This is usually available from pharmacists and is often used to coat non-gold earrings. Wearing a leather watch-strap rather than a metal one may also be more comfortable because it allows the skin to breathe.

Diet

Conventional medical opinion says that diet has little relevance to psoriasis, but most natural therapists disagree. Chapter 7 discusses diet and what you can do to help your skin.

Exercise

Regular exercise is not only good for your physical body, it improves your mental state as well. It stimulates the brain to produce *endorphins*, natural pain-killers and relaxants which raise a sense of well-being. Exercise also improves circulation, stimulates the appetite and improves resistance to viruses and infections. It doesn't have to be hyper-strenuous – a brisk walk in the park will do, if taken regularly. Exercise also often provides opportunities to meet new people in less stressful situations, and the versatility of sportswear – T-shirts, long-sleeved leotards, leggings and tracksuits – can give you cover when you need it. Remember, too, that your body needs sunlight to synthesize vitamin D from food. Vitamin D is the basis of one of the newest conventional therapies for psoriasis (*see* page 41).

Surrogate sun

The sun is a natural healer for most people with psoriasis. Except for the unlucky few (less than 10 per cent), a good dose of sunshine can make dramatic changes to their appearance. Some people find the scaly patches disappear completely in the summer months.

It is the ultraviolet B (UVB) rays that bring the benefit, but as these are also the rays that can cause sunburn, don't overdo it. If you live in a country where there's little chance of overdoing it, even in summer, you can buy special UVB lamps for home use. But be warned: the common or garden commercial sunbed is useless as a treatment because it usually emits only tanning UVA rays.

Spending some time with a UVB lamp can ease the embarrassment of stepping onto the beach in your 'winter skin'. Many sufferers face a dilemma: they know the sun is good for them, but are loath to reveal any more of their skin in public than they have to. But if you do use a sunlamp at home, always talk to a specialist first about the correct amount of time to spend under it, and always use goggles. *See* Chapter 7 for more about light treatments.

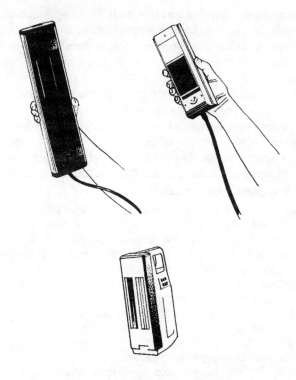

Fig. 2 Examples of UVB lamps suitable for home use

Relationships

It is easy to feel that all other people see of you is a red
raw skin. So it's very important to find ways to counter
those feelings. Otherwise they will undermine your confidence and self-esteem and make it difficult to develop
both friendly and intimate relationships.

The old saying that beauty is not skin deep is still
true; and if you don't dwell on your skin condition, others are not likely to either. It's the person you project

that others see – and if that is a friendly, happy, interesting person, you might be surprised to find that people don't even notice that the skin on your hands or arms is different. The important thing is to reach out to people, not to close down and hide.

And remember, resorting to 'comforters' such as smoking, alcohol and drugs will probably make your skin condition worse, as well as doing little for your long-term well-being. Smoking and alcohol are psoriasis trigger factors for many people, especially women.

Feeling good about yourself

- Accentuate the positive – when you do things well or achieve things, or just have a good day, celebrate with a treat: a glass of wine, new clothes, a day out.
- Take care of your skin, hair and clothes; look for colours and fabrics you feel good in.
- Cultivate a range of interests and get actively involved – don't just read books about them.
- Don't let having a clear skin be your only goal in life – set out to run a marathon, learn Spanish, complete a Thai cooking course, write a poem.
- Use your experience to empathize with other people – everyone has problems and needs to talk sometimes.
- Smile at yourself in the mirror – sounds stupid, but you'll be amazed how, even when you don't feel like it, smiling can lift the spirits.

Psoriasis in children

The first thing a child with psoriasis needs is knowledge. Explain very carefully exactly what psoriasis is in physical terms, how it can come and go, and how what's going on in our lives can affect the skin. Also explain that there are many different kinds of treatment that you can try with them, but be very careful not to show anxiety or frustration if treatments don't work. It is a terrible burden for children to feel it is their fault that you are upset.

It is also important for children to know they are not alone. If a child is the only psoriasis sufferer in the family, a local or national organization may be able to put you in touch with other children who your child could meet or write to. Encourage children to talk to you about how they feel about their skin – not to bottle it up or worry about being misunderstood – and when they are old enough to take some responsibility themselves, suggest they keep a little notebook so that they can be their own detective with things that make their skin react. Find ways to make physical contact and show you love them so that a sore skin doesn't become a barrier between you.

Make sure, too, that teachers, sports instructors and club leaders know and understand the child's skin condition and that they will intervene if he or she is bullied or ostracized. But do this with your child's full knowledge and agreement – there's nothing worse than the surprise attention a child gets when a teacher brings up the subject of psoriasis without any warning.

One of the most difficult things with child sufferers is to stop them scratching. Keep fingernails short, and when the skin itches, suggest they rub it gently rather than using their nails, which will break the skin. Covering lesions with clothing or even bandages at night can help, as does wearing mittens, because children may scratch unthinkingly. But never *ever* be tempted to tie children's hands – it is cruel and psychologically damaging.

Children with extensive psoriasis may need more sleep than other children. The condition causes increased heat- and energy-loss, which can only be restored through sleep. Tiredness will also make the condition worse, and a flare-up accompanied by irritability and crying are tell-tale signs of lack of sleep. Teach your child relaxation tricks – imagining a lovely scene at the beach or in the country on summer holidays, perhaps (*see* page 86 for more ideas).

Gentle herbal teas or cider vinegar (which helps purify the blood) and honey may help them to sleep if they are particularly pent-up.

CHAPTER 5

Conventional treatments and procedures

What your doctor has to offer

Conventional medicine regards psoriasis as 'incurable' because it doesn't know what causes the condition. So conventional treatments tend to work on either suppressing symptoms or easing them as much as possible. The trouble with many conventional approaches is that the treatment is almost as bad as the condition.

- *Topical therapies* (applied directly to the skin) often smell unpleasant, are difficult and messy to use, and stain everything they touch. They frequently have a very limited effect.
- *Systemic therapies* (either swallowed or injected) affect all the body's systems, not just the skin, and are usually designed to reduce the rate of cell production. But they are strong medicine and all have some sort of side-effects, as well as placing a strain on otherwise healthy parts of the body such as the liver, lungs, bones and heart.

What will the doctor do?

Many people with psoriasis never approach their family doctor. In some cases this is because their skin lesions are small and mild, or in an out-of-the-way place and don't bother them, or because they find that they can keep the condition under control with products available from a pharmacy (*see* page 29).

If you cannot control your condition with these products, your family doctor may prescribe other topical therapies. But if your psoriasis is severe and extensive, you may be offered systemic treatments. For these you usually need to see a hospital skin specialist because of the possibility of side-effects.

When you visit your doctor, he or she should assess two things:

- The clinical severity of your condition – that is, how much of your body is involved and how severe the lesions are.
- How bad *you* feel your psoriasis is, and the effect it is having on your life.

The doctor may use a 'body map' to indicate where and how big your patches are, so that any changes can be easily seen. They may ask you what most upsets you about your psoriasis. This is taken into consideration when they work out the type of therapy to offer.

It is important to get the doctor to explain fully the risks and benefits of each of the treatments suggested. Because there is such a wide variety, you need as much information as possible in order to make the right choice. Some therapies can cause toxic effects in otherwise healthy organs; for example, *retinoids* have been linked in research with non-cancerous brain tumours (pseudo-tumour cerebri) and musculo-skeletal and cardiac problems, *methotrexate* may have liver and lung effects, and *cyclosporin A* can affect the blood and kidneys.

Treatments for mild and moderate psoriasis

As mentioned above, many people control their own psoriasis by using products such as skin softening and moisturizing creams lotions and bath oils. These can help control scaling, are easy to use and are usually free of side-effects, but they only act on the surface and cannot do anything about the underlying disease process.

A doctor will usually prescribe one or other of a number of topical treatments. These often contain ingredients such as coal tar, *dithranol* or *corticosteroids*, which are described below. Another relatively new treatment is the vitamin D-based *calcipotriol*.

You can increase the effectiveness of some topical creams by covering the affected areas overnight with a plastic bag or cling film. This helps open the pores and increases the amount of the drug which penetrates the skin. But do not do this with topical steroids without your doctor's approval: you could overdose and damage your skin.

Ultraviolet B radiation can also improve the effectiveness of topical treatments, but this too must be done under expert supervision. Some people respond to one topical treatment better than another, and if one doesn't work, the doctor will often suggest trying another before moving on to more aggressive treatments.

Coal tar

Coal tar is an old therapy, first used in 1925. It is considered very safe and comes in a variety of forms which are put directly onto the skin. It works by reducing itching and inflammation and helping to thin down the rough lesions that develop with psoriasis. Unfortunately it is most effective in its messiest form – combined with petroleum jelly or made into a sticky paste.

Because it can stain clothing and bed linen, coal tar is best used at night under bandages or plastic bags. Pre-impregnated bandages are cleaner and can be worn for a week or so, but still draw unwanted attention. However refined, more visually acceptable ways of using tar are much less effective.

Dithranol

Dithranol is a synthetic substance derived from the drug *chrysarobin*, which reduces cell turnover. This, too, has been around for a long time – some 65 years – and can be more effective than coal tar, though is equally unpleasant to use. It stains skin, baths and clothes with brownish-purple patches which won't wash out, and great care is needed to ensure it doesn't get on unaffected skin where it can cause irritation and soreness.

Dithranol was originally used as an overnight therapy and affected parts of the body had to be covered by bandages. Now, however, it can be used as 'short-contact therapy' – the patient applies the paste for 15 to 45 minutes every 24 hours, then washes it off, making the treatment easier to bear and no less effective.

Topical corticosteroids

The natural steroids produced by the body regulate many of our chemical processes, including our reaction to stress. *Corticosteroids* are a synthetic version of these substances and are produced in lotions and creams.

Steroid preparations are undoubtedly effective in many cases. On the plus side, they reduce inflammation, relieve symptoms and allow damaged skin to heal; they are also clean and easy to use and don't smell. Their main problem is that they do not get rid of the psoriasis. As soon as you stop taking them, the plaques return – in some unfortunate cases, worse than before – and stopping them suddenly can trigger other forms of psoriasis.

There is a danger of side-effects if corticosteroids are used continuously. The chemicals in topical creams and lotions are easily absorbed into the bloodstream. With over-use they can damage the skin's collagen content and cause it to become thin, fragile and prone to damage. Children are particularly at risk from steroid over-use because their skin is thinner and more absorbent. There have also been suggestions that steroids may interfere with growth.

There are other side-effects. Because steroids reduce inflammation by blocking the immune system, they may also interfere with the body's normal healing processes and reduce resistance to infection. They are also greedy consumers of vitamin D, zinc and potassium (which the liver also needs in good quantities to stay healthy) and they trick the body into producing smaller amounts of the natural steroids (including hydrocortisone) that help us deal with stress. Since even many conventional doctors believe that stress is a key player in psoriasis, this is a particularly damaging side-effect.

Because of these effects, steroids are supposed to be used for only short periods. But as psoriasis users know that as soon as they stop their skin condition will return, many continue to use corticosteroid preparations for years – and, indeed, are given repeat prescriptions for them.

Vitamin D therapy

Calcipotriol is the newest of the prescribable topical treatments. It is made from a form of vitamin D, and though it is not clear exactly how it works, it appears to slow the development of *keratinocytes* – the cells that make up the top horny layer of the epidermis. Like steroids, it does not stain or smell and, so far, does not appear to have the systemic side-effects associated with steroids, even when used on up to 40 per cent of the body.

Recent studies have shown it can be used for an unlimited time with no long-lasting side-effects as long as no more than 100g is used per week. It can, however, cause skin irritation in some people.

Scalp treatments

All scalp treatments come as either lotions or shampoos. Coal tar shampoo is most commonly used for mild or moderate conditions. But in more severe cases, the concoctions become more messy and complex. The hospital pharmacist may prepare an *unguentum cocois* compound, which contains coal tar, salicylic acid and sulphur to remove the scale, mixed in a coconut-oil base. The coconut oil melts at skin temperature and both moisturizes and helps spread the ingredients through the hair to the affected skin.

Stronger medicines

If your psoriasis is more severe, you will usually be referred to a specialist unit where there will be a variety of treatment options. The rates of success vary, depending on the individual, and almost all of the treatments have some immediate or long-term side-effects. Deciding whether to carry on with a treatment may well be a matter of weighing up which causes you more distress – the treatment or the psoriasis. Your doctor will want to see you regularly and may need to do regular blood tests to ensure the treatment is not causing internal damage. And with most systemic therapies it is important that men and women sufferers take steps to prevent pregnancy, both while on the therapy and for some time afterwards, because of the risks of deformity to the baby.

Light therapies

Light therapy for psoriasis splits into two types: ultravi-olet A (UVA) and ultraviolet B (UVB). UVA, the tanning ray in sunshine, can do little for psoriasis sufferers by itself, but is quite successful when combined with the drug psoralens (*see* below). UVB is the part of the light spectrum that produces the biological effects of being in the sun – skin reddening and burning. But when used carefully, UVB is also the ray that, by itself, can have positive effects on psoriasis.

PUVA

In ancient times, Egyptians afflicted with skin conditions used to eat a herb that grew beside the Nile and then lie in the sun to cure themselves. PUVA (which stands for *psoralens* plus ultraviolet A light) is the modern version of the Nile treatment.

Patients take a tablet of psoralens (a skin-sensitizing agent) and then lie under specially designed UVA-emit-ting lamps. Twice-weekly treatments in the hospital out-patients department over a period of one or two months are usually needed, and doses are carefully controlled to ensure against 'sunburn'. Patients also have to wear glasses to protect their eyes, both under the lamp and for up to 24 hours afterwards.

PUVA is many doctors' first-choice treatment for dif-ficult psoriasis because it is thought to be the least toxic of all the internal treatments. It can give good results, clearing the skin in up to 90 per cent of patients in four to six weeks, but some people suffer nausea, stomach pain, headaches and lethargy. There may also be an increased risk of skin cancer if PUVA is used over long periods.

One way of avoiding some of the side-effects is 'bath PUVA'. This involves bathing in a psoralens solution for 15 minutes then hopping rapidly under a UVA lamp (the psoralens effect falls away quickly once you are out of the water). This method can considerably reduce these side-effects, but it does take longer to clear the skin.

UVB

Many dermatology units around the world now use UVB radiation, either by itself or to increase the benefits of the topical treatments described above. Many units are open long hours so that patients can visit for treatment on their way to or from work, enabling them to lead as normal a life as possible. Home UVB units make the treatment much more convenient, but users need counselling to ensure they know all the safeguards. And be warned, therapeutic lamps are designed to emit particular wavelengths of light and are very different from normal commercial sun lamps.

UVB is generally more effective than topical steroids. It has similar results to dithranol and coal tar but is more pleasant to use; and its side-effects are generally milder than PUVA and systemic therapies such as methotrexate (*see* below). Most patients are clear of lesions after about two months of five treatments a week (each lasting between 90 seconds and 15 minutes). On average the skin then stays clear for another two months and shows only mild symptoms for a further two months.

UVB is also the key to the alternative, climate-based therapies described in Chapter 7.

Methotrexate

Methotrexate is a long-standing *cytotoxic* therapy for suppressing psoriasis. It works by killing off cells, and is also used to treat various types of cancer. It is a potent drug and can be very toxic, particularly if taken too frequently or for too long. The build-up of toxins can affect the liver, kidneys and bone marrow, and can irritate the stomach and bowel. Other more immediate side-effects are nausea, stomach pain, mouth ulcers, hair loss, tiredness and depression. Patients also have to be careful of interactions with other substances, especially alcohol, and usually have to see their doctor regularly for blood and liver tests.

Retinoids

Retinoids (*etretinate*, for example) are derived from vitamin A. This treatment is used for very stubborn and severe cases of psoriasis, but, as with other strong treatments, there is a price to pay: the most immediate side-effects are dry irritable eyelids, stuffy nostrils and cracking around the mouth. In fact, many doctors see these signs as an indication that the dose is correct. The skin also becomes fragile, and some users report having to wear soft shoes and be careful not to use their hands strenuously as the skin seems to 'wear out'.

Retinoids are gentler on the liver than methotrexate, but there are concerns about links with heart disease and bone problems. Patients need to have lipid level and liver function tests every six months. Conception must be prevented both during treatment and for up to a year afterwards, because of the drug's damaging effects on the unborn child.

Cyclosporin A

Cyclosporin A works on the basis that psoriasis is a disease caused by a faulty immune system. Its main function is to slow down the T-helper cells; these are thought to be responsible for making the body hypersensitive and are found in excess in psoriatic skin. The one most worrying side effect is kidney damage, and patients are monitored closely for this. Other side-effects include mild liver damage and raised blood pressure.

Treatments for psoriatic arthritis

Treatments for psoriatic arthritis are generally the same as those for other forms of arthritis. If the joints are only mildly inflamed, treatment generally starts with physiotherapy and exercise and anti-inflammatory drugs such as *ibuprofen*. However, as the disease progresses more potent drugs that help slow joint destruction, such as sulphazalazine may be offered.

CHAPTER 6

The natural therapies and psoriasis

Introducing the gentle alternatives

Natural therapies have gained enormously in popularity in recent years. Surveys in Britain carried out since the late 1980s, for example, have consistently shown a growing number of people consulting an alternative therapist and a majority of the population believe these kinds of therapies should be provided free on the National Health Service. Similar findings have been reported in North America, Australia and elsewhere.

Conventional doctors are also increasingly more open to the use of alternative therapies. In Britain, again, about a third of family doctors have some training in a natural therapy – most often acupuncture, osteopathy or homoeopathy – and a growing number of hospitals and health centres either offer services or advise people on where to go.

Many natural therapists focus on reducing anxiety as the pathway to good health. They believe that if the body is anxious and stressed it cannot function properly, and if one area malfunctions it has a knock-on effect on other areas. This makes the natural or 'complementary' approach particularly appropriate for psoriasis sufferers: even if their condition is not 'caused' directly by stress, psoriasis itself certainly causes stress which makes the condition worse.

Why go to a natural therapist?

People turn to natural medicine for different reasons. Many start looking for other solutions after years of conventional therapy has failed. According to a British survey carried out in 1993, three out of four people who visit natural therapists go with problems conventional medicine has failed to fix. Another survey of patients visiting a British natural health centre found most had a long-standing problem – on average, nine years.

Some people try alternative therapies as a last shot before starting a conventional therapy that may involve strong drugs and unpleasant side-effects. Other people simply prefer the different approach of alternative practitioners, who tend to spend more time with their clients.

These days great emphasis is put on looking after our own health. We are encouraged to eat healthily, exercise, watch ourselves for 'lumps and bumps'. As a result, many of us expect to be involved if we become ill; we do not want to be fobbed off with a prescription. So some people choose a natural therapist because they like to talk about what might be the best approach for them, and they like the time the therapist spends with them and the feeling that they are considered as a whole person rather than just a collection of symptoms.

What is natural therapy?

While alternative or natural medicine takes many forms, almost all therapies share the following principles:

● They work 'holistically' – that is, they treat you as a whole being, composed of mind, body and spirit, and not just as a bundle of symptoms or a machine that's gone wrong. Therapists take into account your personality, emotions and lifestyle, as well as external influences like surroundings and social relationships.

- They believe good health comes from being in a state of emotional, physical, mental and spiritual balance, and that imbalance is what makes for 'dis-ease' and illness. In some therapies this balance also has to do with a 'life-force' or energy which is thought to run throughout the body and the universe as a whole. In Chinese medicine this is called *chi* or *qi* (pronounced 'chee') and takes the form of two opposing forces (*yin* and *yang*) which symbolize the opposites of life – feminine and masculine, positive and negative, gentleness and strength, intellect and passion, cold and hot, and so on. In India this force is known as *prana*, and in Japan as *ki*. Natural therapists use a variety of ways – remedies, needles, massage and meditation – to activate or direct this life-force.

- They believe the body has a natural ability to heal itself and that the function of treatment is to help our own healing powers. Many see symptoms as the result of the body's attempts to cure itself and believe that rather than trying to 'cure' the symptoms, treatment should work on the root cause of the problem. Because of this you might go away with a prescription that appears to have no connection with what you consulted the therapist for.

- They consider that the kind of person you are – your personality, emotions and circumstances – is at least as important as the condition you have when it comes to deciding on your treatment. This means that two people with the same illness may receive different medication.

Diagnosing the problem

Natural therapists place a lot of importance on your 'history'. They usually want to go into a great deal of detail and may ask you about your diet and habits, lifestyle, family and even events in your childhood. But you will also come across some other techniques.

Acupuncturists, for example, are likely to take your pulses – all 12 of them. Each pulse looks after a different system (the waste disposal system or the reproductive system, say) and its beat gives the therapist information about the energy levels there. Pulses are also sometimes used to test for food allergy. A change in beat when you eat or come close to a food suggests an allergy. Some therapists use a special machine called Vega, which tests by monitoring changes in acupuncture points. Also popular, particularly in Europe, is a similar device called the Mora therapy unit (*see* box).

Another alternative method of diagnosis is iridology, where the practitioner studies the markings on your iris (the coloured part of the eye). Though the evidence to date is unconvincing, these are thought by some to give a detailed picture of your past, present, and even future health. Other therapists use a pendulum – usually a crystal or stone on a chain – and arrive at their diagnosis by interpreting its movements when it is swung over a part of the body, or even over a photograph of the person or a diagram of the organ. This is known as 'medical dowsing' or 'radiesthesia'.

Therapists may use 'muscle-testing' – sometimes called applied kinesiology (AK) – to assess weakness in some area of the body. For this they first measure your resistance by pushing against your upheld hand or arm. They may then ask you to hold a suspect food in one hand, or a damaging thought in your mind, while they push again. The difference in your resistance guides the diagnosis. Some therapists also use this method to decide whether the medicine they give you is the right one.

Mora therapy

Mora therapy attempts to identify weakness and imbalance in patients' physical organs and systems by measuring the electromagnetic field around them. This is done by taking a reading from a probe placed at the end of each of the energy pathways or *meridians* that are thought to criss-cross the body (*see* page 101).

The dial on a Mora therapy unit reads from one to 100; if a reading from each pathway were 50, this would indicate that the patient's body was in perfect working order. A swing one way or the other from this balance points to a weakness or degeneration in the organ served by that pathway. This information can guide therapists to the possible root cause of a symptom such as skin inflammation in psoriasis and help them select the right combination of remedies.

The Alternative Centre in London (a clinic that has pioneered holistic treatments for psoriasis) found that Mora testing showed psoriasis patients to have multiple imbalances. In the 126 patients tested, 115 had an imbalance in the lungs, 126 imbalance in the colon, 124 imbalance in the digestive system and 125 imbalances in the liver and kidneys.

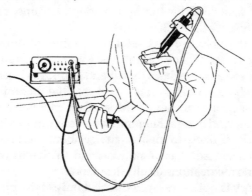

Fig. 3 A Mora therapy unit

What is it like seeing a natural therapist?

Although they all share, more or less, the beliefs already described, you are likely to come across a great variety of people in natural therapy – the range is far wider, it seems, than among family practitioners. Dress may range from the formal and conventional to the informal and even quite wacky.

Equally the premises can be very different. While some natural therapists present a 'brass plaque' image – working in a clinic with a receptionist and an aura of brisk efficiency – others may greet you and treat you in their living room, surrounded by plants and domestic clutter. Remember, though, image is no guarantee of expertise – you are just as likely to find a good, fully qualified therapist working at home and dressed in jeans as in a formal clinic dressed in a suit. (*See* Chapter 10 for how to find and choose a therapist you can trust.)

The principles of natural therapists do lead to approaches that may be different to those you are used to with your family doctor. For example:

- Consultations usually take longer. The initial visit rarely lasts less than an hour, though treatment visits usually last around 30 minutes.
- You are likely to be asked a wide range of questions about yourself: your emotions, job, family, relationships, social life, what you eat and drink, and sleeping and relaxation habits. This is so that the therapist can form a proper understanding of all the elements of your life and assess them in relation to your problem.
- Therapy is likely to involve advice about your lifestyle – diet, exercise, sleep, emotions, and so on – as well as specific medications or physical therapy.
- Therapy is not necessarily directed only at the problem you came with, but may encompass any aspects the therapist feels are out of balance.

- Treatments may take longer to work because their aim is to treat the root of the problem rather than offer rapid symptom relief. This means you may need to allow more time – and have more patience – with natural therapies than conventional medicine, and to have an understanding from the beginning of the way the therapy works so that you do not become disillusioned.

- You are generally expected to be actively involved in the healing process and start to take more responsibility for your health. Many natural approaches require you to change things in your life.

- You will most likely have to pay separately for any remedies prescribed and therapists may well sell you these from their own stocks. They may also charge you an hourly rate for their time – though many therapists offer reduced rates for people who genuinely cannot afford the full fee.

Healing crisis

Most practitioners following holistic systems will warn you that your symptoms are likely to get slightly worse before they get better, and even that old symptoms might reappear. This is called the 'healing crisis' and occurs because many of the systems of alternative medicine work by jolting the body's own defences into fighting again and throwing off the toxins or infections causing the illness. Often this is done quite violently, which is why more symptoms are produced. But the crisis is usually brief and, though sometimes uncomfortable, is considered a good sign that healing energies have started to counteract the illness.

Does natural medicine work?

Plenty of individuals have stories of the success of alternative therapies. But solid 'scientific' proof is harder to come by, although the body of evidence for many treatments is growing year by year. Researchers at Glasgow University in Scotland, for example, have proved the effectiveness of homoeopathic remedies for hayfever and arthritis using the same stringently controlled tests used by pharmaceutical companies. But there are particular difficulties in testing alternative medicine in conventional ways.

Scientific trials usually compare a group of patients who are given one standardized treatment with a group given a *placebo* or fake treatment. But in alternative medicine, the same treatment would rarely be appropriate for a group of people because therapists take all sorts of features into account, not just the symptoms. Plus many therapies – hypnosis, meditation and acupuncture, for example – do not involve medication at all and so cannot be replaced by a fake medication.

It is also important to remember that psoriasis is a chronic disease which by its nature, comes and goes. So if you happen to start a therapy just when a flare-up is beginning to weaken, the treatment may appear to be working fantastically when, in fact, your skin would have cleared up anyway.

Nevertheless, two thirds of the people surveyed in one British natural health centre said they had experienced some improvement with natural treatments. And those who had faith in the methods were more likely to benefit. It may be that alternative therapies are more effective with the kind of long-term ailments often described as the 'diseases of civilization' – stress, depression, migraine, rheumatism and skin conditions – while orthodox medicines are better for 'emergencies', when rapid relief from acute symptoms is needed.

What do doctors think of natural medicine?

The attitude of doctors to natural medicine ranges from complete scepticism to enthusiastic use. While a small proportion dismiss it as 'quackery' and another small (but increasing) number are training themselves in techniques such as herbalism, acupuncture, hypnosis and homoeopathy, the vast majority are in the middle – broadminded about some approaches, less convinced about others, but prepared to concede that natural therapies generally do no harm.

The most common reservations about natural medicine are:

- the lack of conventional research into the effects of many treatments
- the inability to explain how therapies work in conventional scientific and medical terms
- the possibility of missing serious disease if patients consult non-medically trained therapists before seeing a doctor
- the lack of regulation regarding qualifications and lack of safeguards for patients in most alternative disciplines

There are, of course, precautions to take when choosing a therapist, even after you begin the consultation. These are explained in Chapter 10.

CHAPTER 7

Diet and environmental therapies

Using food, water and sunshine to heal your skin

Many alternative practitioners believe food and the substances we inadvertently consume in the air we breathe and the water we drink, play a major role in psoriasis. Fatty foods, high-protein food, sweet stuffs, alcohol, chemicals from food additives and pollution all put stress on the liver and digestive system, they say. More conventional physicians tend not to agree that diet is so important, but this is one area where, with care, you can test the theory for yourself.

Why does it matter what you eat?

It stands to reason that what you put into your digestive system will affect the way it functions. When food is hard to digest, it clogs the works and may not get properly broken down. With some of the things we swallow, the liver has to work very hard to extract what the body needs and to dispose of the rest.

High-protein foods are particularly hard to digest, according to nutritionists. To break them down bacteria in the intestine have to produce an army of toxic compounds known as *polyamines*. But studies have shown that polyamines also force cells to increase the speed at which they divide, which is what happens to skin cells in psoriasis.

Liver overload is another factor. The liver has huge reserves and people who have part of their liver removed or whose liver is damaged through illness, stress or alcohol, can recover – given time. However, what the liver cannot cope with is constant overloading with toxins, especially if it is in a weakened state. Fatty foods, red meat, alcohol and food additives create their own burden of harmful bacteria as they make their slow way through the system. Yeast infections such as candidiasis or 'candida' (which is helped by high-sugar diets) also produce chemicals that encourage cell division and proponents of this theory add that nowadays we are also subject to a constant bombardment of toxic substances from external sources such as agricultural sprays and other environmental pollutants.

When the liver becomes overloaded, it leaves toxins circulating in the bloodstream and the body has to try to eliminate them in other ways – through the skin, for example.

Furthermore, therapists involved in naturopathy, one of the alternative disciplines that puts great emphasis on good diet, believe that people with psoriasis have thinner gut walls as a result of problems such as liver and kidney damage, constipation, food allergy, bacterial infection, even immunization. This means toxins can pass more easily though the gut walls instead of being contained and disposed of safely.

High vegetable content, low-protein diet

It is often said that people eating a typical 'Western' diet are overfed but undernourished. They eat too much of the wrong foods (animal fats, salt, sugar, processed and junk foods) and too little of the right ones. Basic advice for psoriasis sufferers from nutritional therapists is simple.

Cut down on:

- high-protein foods
- acidic foods
- processed and refined products like white flour
- highly spiced and seasoned dishes
- all sweet foods made with sugar

Eat lots of:

- fresh fruit
- vegetables
- natural grains
- legumes (peas and beans)

These all provide plenty of vitamins, minerals and dietary fibre and encourage the waste disposal system to work effectively.

Many nutritional therapists advise avoiding red meat, dairy products and saturated fats completely and eating as many foods as possible raw. Some naturopaths say that yellow and green foods – melon, soybean, saffron tea, carrot juice and seaweeds – are particularly beneficial in the long term, while Chinese medicine recommends avoiding all red foods because they see

---

Eating to help your skin

- Eat plenty of fruits and vegetables.
- Eat more 'oily' fish – mackerel, sardines, salmon, pilchards and herrings.
- Cut down animal fats, particularly dairy products.
- Eat less red meat.
- Avoid heavily processed and refined foods.
- Cut down on sugar and sweet foods.
- Cut down on alcohol and stop smoking.
- Take a fish-oil supplement and a multi-vitamin which includes zinc, vitamin A and vitamin B complex.

psoriasis as a 'red' or 'fire' condition. This applies not only to food of that colour but to food such as chillies and hot spices that create 'fire' in the body. Foods that are difficult to digest also overheat the body.

Food allergies

Although food allergies have not been as strongly linked to psoriasis as they have been to other skin diseases such as eczema, allergic reactions do produce toxins which stress the digestive system just as much as those from other sources. Allergies can prevent the stomach properly absorbing foods and stop nutrients getting into the bloodstream. Even where the blood is chock-full of nutrients, toxins absorbed from the environment may stop the body making full use of them.

Suspect allergy foods for psoriasis sufferers include excess animal fats, acid foods, sugars, spices, salt, stimulants such as alcohol, tea and coffee, and sugary soft drinks.

The way to find out if a food is affecting your skin is to avoid it for several days during a flare-up and then observe the result. If you notice any difference at all, persist for longer. But it is important to remember that psoriasis is a chronic disease and has a natural pattern of flare-ups and clear periods. To identify whether a particular food truly has an effect you may need to avoid and then re-introduce it several times to be sure that the effect is not part of the pattern of the disease.

A more extreme version of this technique is an *exclusion* or *elimination* diet. These diets can be used if avoiding the common allergens has produced no result. They involve eating the most limited, bland and boring selection of food (a classic one is boiled water, lamb, rice and peeled pears) until symptoms settle down (usually about three weeks), then adding in other foods one at a time and recording any changes in symptoms. Any exclusion diet must be carried out under skilled supervision because it can dangerously deplete the body of nutrients.

There are several problems with exclusion diets. They can lead to temporary flare-ups of the allergy or unpleasant and confusing withdrawal symptoms. They can cause new sensitivities because non-restricted foods are eaten in much greater quantities than normal, and they don't always identify the allergy even if it is there, because it can take time for the effect of an allergen to build up. Most conventional doctors put little store in these diets as a result.

Detoxification

Some studies have shown that going through a *detoxification* process to get rid of the accumulated toxins before plunging into a new diet can improve the results. This usually means fasting for two or three days – eating nothing and drinking only fruit and vegetable juices or herb teas – then moving on to eating fruits and gradually adding in other foods from your new diet over a period of days or even weeks.

Some people say treatments such as colonic irrigation, where the intestine is gently flushed out with warm water, help the detoxification process, although most doctors are very sceptical.

It is important not to fast, start a limited diet or start taking supplements without advice from a trained nutritionist. You should also have a medical check-up to make sure you are not suffering from any illness that could become worse if you are in a weakened state. Remember also that some nutritional supplements may interact with prescribed medicines: for example, high doses of vitamin C can reduce the effect of drugs taken for heart conditions. So check before you start.

Dairy products

Some practitioners believe dairy products are the root of all evil when it comes to psoriasis. They say they are hard to digest and take a long time to pass through the body, leaving plenty of time for toxins to build up. The fat content sticks to the lining of the stomach, preventing nutrients passing into the bloodstream and depriving other organs of minerals they need. Cow's milk is also thought to cause overproduction of mucus, and substantial numbers of people are thought to be allergic to lactose (milk sugar). Allergy to dairy products has been linked to many other conditions – eczema, asthma, migraine, joint and blood disease, and hyperactivity – but most evidence linking it with psoriasis is anecdotal.

Alcohol

Drinking alcohol almost certainly makes psoriasis worse. Some studies show that people with psoriasis tend to drink more than other people, although that does not mean alcohol causes the condition. It may well be that psoriasis sufferers turn to alcohol because they are miserable and lonely.

Jacqui's story

Jacqui was a healthfood enthusiast. She never ate refined or processed foods; she took vitamin and mineral supplements, and exercised frequently. Her only 'vice' was an occasional glass of red wine in the evening. And if she drank a glass several nights in a row, her psoriasis would flare up. She wasn't a heavy drinker by any means, but her liver was weak enough to react to even the gentle overload of a glass of wine. The solution, at least was simple.

Supplementing your diet

Many nutritional therapists advise people with psoriasis to supplement their diet with a variety of vitamins, minerals and oils. Some of this advice has evidence to back it up, though in most cases it has not been proved to the satisfaction of medical doctors.

Remember supplements are chemicals in their own right and can cause just as many problems of balance as chemicals consumed by accident. So take advice on which supplements should be taken together and don't exceed the prescribed dose.

Fish oil and evening primrose oil

Fish oils are thought to be beneficial because of their high content of *eicosapentaenoic acid* (EPA). This is one of a set of compounds called *essential fatty acids*. Some nutritionists think psoriasis is caused when the body's levels of these essential fatty acids are out of kilter: there is too much of one type and not enough of another.

Studies have found the skin of psoriasis sufferers contains high levels of *leucotrienes*. These compounds (which cause inflammation) are manufactured by the essential fatty acid called *arachidonic acid*. This is found exclusively in animal fats and is the main reason why nutritionists suggest people with psoriasis should cut their intake of animal fats to a bare minimum. They also suggest taking fish oil because the EPA it contains appears to knock out arachidonic acid, thus slowing down the production of leucotrienes and reducing inflammation.

The case for evening primrose oil is that its essential fatty acid – *gammalinoleic acid* – stokes up the levels of the 'good' fatty acids by preventing them changing into arachidonic acid.

A Danish study of 17 psoriasis patients treated with a combination of fish and evening primrose oils, for example, found that after four months two patients had virtually no symptoms, eight showed moderate improvement, four showed mild improvement, and in three patients the treatment had no effect. However, other studies have shown little benefit.

But studies into coal tar, used for years as therapy for psoriasis, seem to back up the theory because coal tar appears to increase levels of the 'good' fatty acids in the body.

Zinc

The mineral zinc is involved with controlling inflammation and activating the immune system. Many studies have shown zinc can help skin conditions and some practitioners recommend taking high doses (up to 30–40 milligrams a day) for long periods. However, taking zinc alone can deplete other minerals such as copper. It is more sensible to take a multi-vitamin tablet containing no more than 15–20 milligrams of elemental zinc.

Fumaric acid

Fumaric acid forms on your skin when you are exposed to sunlight, but psoriasis sufferers seem to need a very long time in the sun to produce this substance. Trials of psoriasis patients who take fumaric acid supplements have produced good results, with eight in ten patients showing improved skin and six in ten clearing their psoriasis completely, provided they kept taking it. But slight changes in kidney and liver function were also observed, so it's important to take the therapy under professional supervision.

Also, this therapy requires patience – it can take up to three months for any effect to show. The dose gradually increases, starting with one 500 milligram capsule a day for the first two weeks, two for the next two weeks, and so on, up to a maximum of seven capsules daily.

Some patients notice a warm tingly feeling in the skin on the neck and shoulders which lasts about 15 minutes. Therapists say this means the desired reaction is taking place. After the first 14 days, the skin may become more itchy and the hands and feet may swell slightly. Again, this is supposed to show the therapy is working, but talk to a therapist if it lasts more than a few days. When the skin has substantially cleared, the dose can be reduced to one or two capsules daily.

Other supplements

Many therapists believe that although we now have far greater variety in our diet, the stressful conditions we live in and the way we prepare our food means that we are still deficient in certain important vitamins and minerals. The following are commonly thought to help psoriasis:

- vitamin A – 10,000iu three times a day for six days a week to slow the rate of cell division
- vitamin B complex – 100 milligrams twice a day with meals to combat organ damage from stress
- vitamin D – 400iu a day (not really a vitamin but a hormone made by the body from sunlight; now a component in conventional treatments for psoriasis and associated with the effectiveness of climatotherapy (*see* page 69)
- Spirulina – an algae product rich in trace minerals
- tissue salts – *silica, nat sulph, kali phos, ferr phos, calc sulph*

Naturopathy

The broad approach and general philosophy of naturopathy is said to be particularly effective for skin disorders. Naturopaths use a complex mixture of nutritional therapy, homoeopathy (*see* page 96), botanical or herbal medicine, spinal manipulation, hydrotherapy, and physical and mental exercise. They emphasize good nutrition and exercise, living naturally and thinking positively. Good therapists are usually well regarded by the medical profession.

First-line therapy for skin conditions is usually dietary change based on information the therapist gains by asking detailed questions, not only about what you eat but about how you think and feel, your relationships, activities and lifestyle. You may be asked to fast for three to five days – either on water or on fruit or vegetable juices – to detoxify your system. This will be followed by recommendations on long-term diet along the lines described in the diet section above.

Naturopaths believe illness results when a person's 'vital force' is weakened or out of balance and that the cause is most often a deficient lifestyle – too much stress, food loaded with chemicals, environmental pollution, and not enough fresh air and exercise.

They also believe that the body will always try to heal itself and regain its harmony. Rather than knock out symptoms with drugs, they prefer to use symptoms to identify the underlying cause of problems and then help the body to repair itself. If the body can heal broken bones, they reckon it can probably deal quite adequately with other disorders, given half a chance.

Nutritional therapy

Nutritional therapists believe that most people, even those who appear to eat well, have nutritional deficiencies due to an unbalanced diet, food allergies, early life events such as childhood illnesses, or stressful life situations, and environmental stress. They focus on identifying and correcting the deficiencies by concentrating on three main areas:

- food or environmental allergies
- toxic overload resulting from exposure to heavy metals and chemicals in the environment
- reduced ability of digestive systems and organs to deal with toxins

Therapists often use special blood tests and hair analyses to identify vitamin and mineral deficiencies, as well as taking very detailed personal information. Treatment then takes the form of dietary changes and supplementa-

---

Dr Ann's story

Dr Ann, a family doctor with psoriasis, visited a nutritional therapist after trying to devise a diet to control her skin. She had tried eliminating certain foods but it seemed just about everything caused a flare-up. The therapist diagnosed a severely disturbed liver; almost 50 different food groups were identified as poisons that the liver was unable to break down.

Dr Ann was put on a *rotation* diet, designed to reduce exposure to any food toxin and give the liver a chance to recover. She could eat, for example, rice on Monday, millet on Tuesday, lentils on Wednesday, and so on. The foods chosen were those that caused the least upset.

After about six weeks on this very restricted diet, her skin was much improved and she was able to take up a more lenient diet, though still being careful not to overload the liver. After six months, Dr Ann's liver had recovered and her skin was clear – and stayed clear as long as she stayed away from three or four foods that were finally identified as the key culprits.

tion. Detoxification (*see* page 60) is often used as a first step, and the diets that follow can be quite radical initially. However, therapists are trained to motivate and counsel and most people find it easier to follow the regimens once they start seeing results.

Many well-conducted studies have shown nutritional medicine to be of benefit, particularly to those with chronic illness. An audit of 300 National Health Service patients in England treated by a nutritional therapist between 1990 and 1993 found 54 per cent of patients with skin conditions reported 'definite lasting improvement'.

Clinical ecology

Clinical ecologists believe disorders such as psoriasis result from our reactions to the environment we live in. They say that modern lifestyles are a far cry from the primitive conditions to which humans are biologically tuned, and the toxic substances we now encounter in the environment – lead in water pipes, food additives, pesticides and industrial pollutants – have outpaced our bodies' ability to adapt.

Though we can cope with this onslaught of stress and pollution for a while, at a certain point it becomes too much and the body becomes 'sensitized' to whatever chemicals are most prevalent, and collapses in one way or another. This often happens when the immune system has been weakened by viral infections such as flu or glandular fever.

Clinical ecologists trace many 'modern' ailments – obesity, asthma, psoriasis, eczema, hay fever, migraine, arthritis and inflammatory bowel disease – back to this increased sensitivity. Sensitivity may not always be the same as a proper allergy, where the immune system responds as if attacked from outside. It may be that environmental pollution makes extra demands on the body's nutrient levels, leaving it lacking in the minerals and vitamins vital for health. This may lead to gut abnormalities which stop food being broken down properly; again, this denies the body all the nutrients it needs, and which you think you are giving it through the food you eat. Nevertheless many patients respond when their sensitivity is treated in the same way as an allergy – that is by identifying the substance that is causing the problem and then trying to avoid it.

Sometimes a person may have what's called 'masked sensitivity' where symptoms caused by multiple sensitivities gradually appear over time, each one making it easier for another to develop as the body's defences are weakened. When influences such as stress or overwork are added, the body becomes unable to maintain the fight.

As it is not always easy to discover exactly what an individual is reacting to, clinical ecologists employ a range of specialized tests, including:

- allergen tests – an allergen is either placed on the skin on a sticky patch or injected under the skin to see if a reaction occurs
- RAST tests – the blood is scanned for certain antibodies
- cytotoxic tests – the white cells in a blood sample are exposed to suspected allergens
- pulse tests – recording the pulse beat before and at intervals after eating a suspect food
- vega tests – recording electrical currents in the body at specific acupuncture points

Treatment is usually a mixture of manipulating the diet to avoid the offending substance and allow the body to become desensitized, and mineral and vitamin supplements which aim to counteract the imbalances caused by high demand. The problem is that it can be very difficult to avoid substances in the air and water – though practitioners can advise how to lessen the effect of pollution by, for example, taking antioxidant vitamins.

Conventional doctors are often highly sceptical of both the testing methods of clinical ecologists and their treatments, and so far there is little scientific evidence to back them up. Nevertheless, some people believe the benefits are sometimes little less than miraculous.

Climatotherapy

The environment does not always work against us, however. *Climatotherapy* – the use of sunshine, spring waters and mineral-rich mud – has achieved some of the most convincing and long-lasting effects on psoriasis.

The Dead Sea 'Cure'

The Dead Sea, lying between Israel and Jordan, has one of the best reputations of any psoriasis treatment – either complementary or conventional. Large studies by international dermatologists show that between 85 and 90 per cent of psoriasis sufferers have either clear or significantly improved skin after spending three to four weeks in one of the clinics there. One study reported that patients' symptoms stayed away for up to eight and a half months on average, while others have found shorter times – between three and six months. And when symptoms do start to recur, most patients find they are milder. Studies of people with psoriatic arthritis have found that up to 75 per cent are free of joint symptoms after four weeks of Dead Sea treatment.

Explanations for this success involve a combination of factors, all based on the area's unusual climate.

The Dead Sea – so named because it has ten times the mineral content of other sea waters (virtually nothing can live in it) – is the lowest spot on earth. It is 400 metres below sea level and as a result has an extra layer of atmosphere. As well as having high atmospheric pressure and low humidity, it is one of the driest places on earth, with up to 330 sunny days a year.

All these climatic factors mean the waters of the Dead Sea evaporate very quickly. This creates a unique haze that hangs over the entire region. This haze provides a natural filter for the sun's UVB rays, which are the most beneficial type of ray for psoriasis. But these short UVB rays need to be carefully controlled so as not to burn the skin while also allowing the longer UVA rays which tan rather than burn to get through. One study showed that the sunlight reaching the Israeli town of Beer Sheva, not far from the Dead Sea but sited at the great height of 280 metres above sea level, had four times the burning ability of the sunlight reaching the township of Ein Bokek on the shores of the Dead Sea, nearly 700 metres below.

As sunlight helps improve the skin of the majority of psoriasis sufferers, this unique climate means they can expose their skin for far longer without fear of sunburn.

Another characteristic of this magical haze is that it contains large amounts of bromine, a mineral known for its calming effect on the nervous system, and used in many sedative drugs. The Dead Sea itself contains 50 times more bromine than other oceans and 15 times more magnesium, which is known for its anti-allergic influence on the skin and lungs.

Plus, the air in the Dead Sea region is richer in oxygen levels than anywhere else in the world. There is virtually no pollution or allergens in the air and the very low humidity increases the metabolic activity of the body, which makes people feel refreshed and invigorated. All of these factors promote the relaxation so vital for psoriasis sufferers.

But it is not only the sun and the air that have a beneficial impact on skin. The water of the Dead Sea itself also helps – and so does the mud. The high mineral content of the Dead Sea water makes it so buoyant that you can sit in it almost as you would sit in an armchair. The water counteracts the weight of the body and allows you to float with no effort. This is particularly beneficial for people with arthritis, including psoriatic arthritis, because the water takes the strain and makes moving the limbs to regain flexibility possible.

The mud reservoirs, which are rich in salts absorbed from the lake and hormonal products from the mud algae, are found near the hot springs at a small settlement called Ein Gedi. There you can slap the mud on, roll in it, or even be wrapped up in it and covered with clingfilm. These treatments appear to be particularly good for people with psoriatic arthritis.

Israeli researchers found 146 psoriatic arthritis sufferers who bathed at the Dead Sea and had mud packs and sulphur baths improved significantly compared with 20 patients who took only the Dead Sea cure.

Whichever way you choose to be exposed to the waters of the Dead Sea, they are thought to act in a variety of therapeutic ways.

Researchers have found that the heat of the water widens blood vessels, speeds up the circulation and brings down blood pressure as well as increasing body temperature. They believe the dissolved chemicals in the water improve the chemical balance of the skin. Also, the heavier weight of the water seems to increase heart activity and encourage deeper breathing – again stimulating relaxation.

Another important element of the 'cure', scientists believe, is the psychological benefit psoriasis sufferers receive from meeting others with the condition and relaxing and socializing with people who understand. As the clinics are all sited in hotels with sports and entertainment facilities, people can get away from a hospital environment and the constant feeling that they are ill, or odd.

A daily therapy of lying in the sun – without fear of insult or comment – bathing in warm buoyant water, and treating the skin to soothing natural treatments, tends to seem like heaven in comparison with life at home.

For most people it takes between three and four weeks of daily therapy to achieve a lasting improvement. Some people report good results after only 14 days, but generally their improvement does not last so long. The success and lasting effect of climate therapies at the Dead Sea place them alongside the more effective pharmacological treatments. An added advantage is that they do not seem to have any adverse side-effects. Some have suggested UVB treatments might increase the risk of skin cancer, but so far there is no evidence of this.

Staying at a Dead Sea resort is not cheap – but it can work out cheaper than innumerable hospital visits and expensive drugs, not to mention the psychological and social effects of long-term care and possible unemployment. Countries such as Denmark, Germany and Austria take the most enlightened view on this and health authorities in those countries now pay for Dead Sea treatments for its citizens out of public funds. In the United States and some parts of Europe (but not Britain) private health insurance companies will often meet claims for this combination of sun, water and mineral-rich muds, or 'climatotherapy'.

Father José's story

Father José had battled with his psoriasis for 24 years, and more than 60 per cent of his skin was affected. He had visited over 20 specialists in Spain, France and Italy. Each visit ended with a prescription which invariably included a steroid-based ointment, vitamin A pills and a horrible-smelling tar ointment.

'All this was naturally accompanied by a hefty bill and a card for another appointment, since psoriasis turns us into perpetual clients,' he says.

Then he read an article on the Dead Sea. The cost seemed high but calculated that he found he was spending at least the cost of the trip on ointments, doctor's appointments and transport. His social security department refunded some of these expenses but the treatments had made no difference. So in 1980 he decided to give the Dead Sea a try.

At Ein Bokek he bathed in the mineral waters and lay naked in the sun for the first time in years. At the end of four weeks, his arms, legs and body had almost returned to normal and there were only a few traces of scales left.

'When I returned home I was really living again. I had not experienced such an improvement in 24 years. The disease left me in peace for two months and when it reappeared in the third month, it was in a much less acute form.'

Father José has returned to Ein Bokek several times and his condition has improved considerably.

'The cortisone (steroid) poisoning of my legs has now almost disappeared and the formation of the cells has slowed up. Since my first day at the Dead Sea I have not returned once to see a dermatologist and I haven't bought a single tube of ointment.'

Michelle's story

Michelle had suffered from psoriasis for 24 years and had tried everything – steroid creams, PUVA, thermal cures, homoeopathy – all to no avail. She also suffered from psoriatic arthritis and had already had two operations on her right knee, with more planned for her left knee.

'I was in complete despair, Israel was my last chance,' she said.

After just a few days at the Dead Sea, her skin condition started to improve, and after two weeks had cleared completely. Even more surprisingly, her joints began to improve to the point where she was once again able to walk normally. The operations on her left knee were postponed indefinitely on her return home, and one year on from the visit, her knees were still improving.

Other 'cure' centres

There are other places to find 'natural' cures apart from Israel. The Blue Lagoon in Iceland, for example, has been said to improve psoriasis – although the water itself comes from a geothermal power station upstream. And thermal springs throughout Europe, particularly in Germany, Austria and Finland, are said to help psoriasis.

The famous bathing pools of Central Anatolia in Turkey, where 'doctor fish' nibble and lick the sufferers' plaques away, are said to be effective – though with all the concerns over transmission of hepatitis and HIV, this is probably not to be recommended.

In Britain, a health spa specializing in Dead Sea treatments, including Dead Sea mud 'wraps' and mineral baths, has opened in Colchester, Essex (*see* Appendix A).

Do-it-yourself

If you cannot get to any of these more exotic locations to bathe, you could try making up your own 'therapeutic waters' based on herbal remedies. One combination is 250 grams (8 ounces) of sea salt, one tablespoonful of cider vinegar, 15 grams (half an ounce) of camomile flowers and a cup of oats. The last two ingredients should be boiled for about five minutes (you might want to put them in a muslin bag rather than having all the bits floating in the bath). Add everything to a bath and soak in this for about 20 minutes – don't use soap or soap substitutes – then dry yourself gently and apply 'chicko' oil (a combination of chickweed, olive and almond oils) to your psoriasis patches. It is best to take these special baths just before bed, and wrap up well afterwards to help the ingredients work in through the pores of the skin.

Real or synthetic Dead Sea salts that you can buy and add to your bath have also been shown to be effective. Epsom salts in the bath can also help stimulate the circulation and eliminate toxins, but don't use them if you are feeling weak or frail. Another alternative is to soak in a bath to which you have added Austrian peat moor bath liquid, a muddy and rather unpleasant-smelling solution which rich in minerals. It, too, is said to help skin conditions such as psoriasis.

CHAPTER 8

Treating mind and emotions

Therapies to help get your mind on your side

For a long time people thought the mind and the body functioned quite separately and that neither affected the other. Under this philosophy, conventional doctors concentrated on treating the symptoms of disease and paid little attention to what was happening to the person.

But, increasingly, research in the field of medical science has discovered what many unconventional therapists have believed instinctively all along – that the health of mind and body are intricately linked and both need to be brought into play to 'cure' ill-health.

There is everyday evidence for this 'mind-body' link: just thinking about sucking a lemon will make your mouth water, for example. And sportspeople are often able to ignore quite serious injuries because their concentration is totally taken up by the game. It is only when the final whistle blows that the mind allows them to feel pain. Another illustration of this link is that people who *believe* they are drinking alcohol behave as if they are drunk, even if their drinks are, in fact, non-alcoholic. This reaction is known as a placebo effect.

Placebo effect

In medicine a *placebo* effect takes place when a person's belief in the treatment or faith in the practitioner is so powerful that it works, whatever it is. Researchers often test the effect of a drug against the effect of a look-alike sugar pill (the placebo) to try to find out the drug's real benefit.

For example, trials studying the effect of morphine, one of the most powerful pain-killing substances available, found 70 per cent of people felt their pain was relieved by one dose of the drug. But 35 per cent of those given a placebo dose also said their pain was eased. This suggests up to half the effect of morphine could be the result of mind-power.

Of course, it then stands to reason that such power can also have an opposite effect and that treatment may not work so well if someone is negative about it or has fears about the practitioner. Many people's blood pressure, for example, leaps up when it is taken by a doctor rather than by someone else – a phenomenon known as 'white coat hypertension'. One possible reason for this is that these people put more importance on – and therefore feel more nervous about – something done by a doctor than by other medical professionals.

Conventional doctors often dismiss the effects of natural medicine as 'just placebo', or feel uneasy about using a therapy whose results cannot be explained by current scientific research methods – even though, as discussed in Chapter 6, it is almost impossible to study natural medicines, in the same way as conventional drug therapy. This seems a little strange, since what could be better than taking 'nothing' and letting the mind do the rest? However, critics of natural medicine point out that patients may be paying a lot for 'nothing'.

Mind chemistry

What has the mind-body link got to do with the skin, you may ask? Well, many alternative practitioners believe the 'dis-ease' of the mind is the root of physical ill-health and that the physical symptoms are there to alert us to the fact that we have not recognized or dealt with certain psychological and emotional factors in our lives. In other words, the skin, they believe, reflects the state of a person's internal emotional and physical health.

Up until recently this theory had been dismissed by many conventional practitioners as hokum. But researchers are starting to find concrete clinical evidence of this mind-body interaction. By studying the make-up of the immune system, the nervous system and the mind, they have discovered that emotions and thoughts can cause specific chemical changes in the body and these changes affect the messages sent to the immune system.

This means that if people are distressed, feel rejected, lonely or under strain, or if they lack confidence or are suppressing emotions of jealousy, dislike or fear, these negative feelings could be interfering with the body's ability to stay in good running order and ward off infection.

On the other hand, this information also suggests that positive attitudes and a constructive frame of mind could do the opposite and have powerful benefits for health. Studies of women with breast cancer, for example, have shown that those who react with spirit, who believe they can fight off the disease – and have strong motivation and support – do far better than those who approach their illness passively or in a state of resignation.

Surveys of people with skin conditions show that more than a third are in a state of psychological distress, which means they are probably circulating negative thoughts. Other studies have found that the skin of over 50 per cent of psoriasis sufferers started to break up for the first time after some stressful event or period in their lives.

Stress

Stress is a perfect example of the way the mind can affect the body. Think about what happens when you are suddenly scared or angry or anxious. Your heart pounds, you get short of breath, you feel hot and sweaty and you want to either hit out or run. Scientists call this perfectly natural physical reaction to something happening in your mind, the 'fight or flight' reaction. It is a basic instinct that has always been evident in man: in prehistoric times the first humans had to react instinctively to their fear immediately and physically if they did not want to be killed or eaten by a large wild beast.

The skin is inseparably involved in the physical reaction to stress. In a human embryo the skin develops from the same cells as the brain, and both are linked into the part of the nervous system that controls involuntary processes such as those needed to fight or flee. These include changing the temperature and moisture levels in the skin.

The problem is that modern life produces so many situations that stimulate a stress reaction: the state of your skin, traffic jams, the washing machine breaking down, lack of work, too much work, a sick child, planning a wedding, an argument with your partner, and so on.

And it's not only high fliers that get stressed out – frustration, boredom and lack of fulfilment in life can be just as stressful as high expectations and deadlines.

Not all stress is bad of course – we need a certain amount to get things done. But it's a fine line between what we need to motivate us and what kicks us over into feelings of anxiety and lack of control. That line is a very individual one, although some research has found that people who suffer from psoriasis have more anxious personalities than the general population and so may be more affected by stress.

Signs of stress

dry mouth	fear
becoming accident prone	anxiety
forgetfulness	frequent visits to the toilet
irritability and quick temper	headaches
tearfulness	palpitations
feelings of frustration	pains in the chest
insomnia	tiredness and lack of energy
constant feeling of tenseness	
inability to relax	

Stress-related conditions

acne	excessive sweating	impotence
angina	hair loss	itching
asthma	herpes	migraine
colitis	high blood pressure	stomach ulcers
eczema	hives	

The vicious circle

People with psoriasis are caught in a vicious circle. As sufferers know only too well, psoriasis is stressful for many reasons:

- its appearance undermines self-esteem and confidence
- its coming and going causes uncertainty and depression
- life seems to be controlled by the condition and its unpleasant treatments
- there is constant worry about how others will react
- there is guilt about how the condition affects others' lives (not being able to work and bring in a pay packet, for example)

Some people feel their skin is a barrier which traps them and makes them helpless to achieve what they want in life. One sufferer smashed all the china in her kitchen after a shopkeeper refused to put her change into her hand. Another stopped playing sport because he was embarrassed to shower with his teammates.

But stress makes psoriasis worse. With a vicious circle like this, it's no wonder that some sufferers sink into despair and anger.

Hidden meanings

Some therapists believe that rather than causing loss of self-esteem, psoriasis is actually the result of a lack of self-esteem. They argue that the body creates a justification for feeling inadequate. So people who feel they are of no importance, or who are shy and introverted and lack confidence when in society, in effect create their own disease as a barrier to hide behind. The greater their fear the thicker the 'suit of armour' becomes.

And strange as it may seem, some people may have reasons for not wanting to get rid of their skin condition – though they might find this hard to admit. Some feel that if it wasn't for their psoriasis they would be ignored; others are scared they would not be able to live up to others' expectations of them and prefer to keep their 'reason' for not succeeding. Both examples, of course, come back to a lack of self-esteem.

Some alternative therapies, therefore, aim at the personality rather than the physical condition. Flower remedies, of which the Bach remedies are the best known (*see* page 93), are an example of this approach.

Psoriasis sufferers may be directed to the willow remedy if they have become resentful and bitter as a result of what they believe was an unfair or unjust set of circumstances. People who are distant and aloof and possibly creating their own 'protective' skin condition may be prescribed water violet.

Seeking help

There are many therapies which aim to break the vicious circle of stress and psoriasis and to foster a more positive outlook on life. One key element in almost all of them is learning how to relax. Relaxing has the opposite effect to stress on our chemical make-up. It blocks the chemicals which stop the immune system from working effectively, lets the body recover and helps build up resistance to physical and mental stresses.

Relaxing seems like it should be the easiest thing in the world – but it isn't. You pace, you worry, you keep trying to find the solution to your various problems and all the time you are breathing in those short, shallow breaths that tell your body that it's under threat. With all this going on, just saying 'relax' is not enough. You need a few tricks to be able to relax when you need to.

An immediate trick is to stop, slow down the breathand on the out-breath slowly count to ten. Concentrate on pushing your stomach muscles out as you breathe in, and pulling them in as you breathe out.

When you have got more time, lie down comfortably somewhere where you won't be disturbed, close your eyes and take a couple of deep sighing breaths through your nose. Then focus on relaxing each part of the body in turn. Start with your toes, clench them tight for ten seconds and then let them flop. Do the same with your whole foot, then your calves, knees, thighs, hips, stomach, fingers, arms, shoulders and neck. Finally, screw up your face tightly and then let it smooth out gently.

Lie still, feeling your whole body softening and melting into the floor, breathe gently and tell yourself that you are totally at peace. Stay like this for at least five minutes. Then open your eyes, stretch, turn on your side and get up slowly. Try and do this twice a day. You may want to try combining it with some of the following mind-power techniques.

Meditation

A lot of people associate meditation with religion or orange-robed followers of Eastern gurus, but it doesn't have to involve either. Meditation simply takes relaxation a step further and tries to slow the mind down for a while to let it recuperate from day-to-day hassles.

There is quite a body of scientific research to back the beneficial effects of daily meditation. It produces measurable changes in brainwave patterns, muscular tension, blood pressure and circulation. It is often used in hospitals to reduce high blood pressure or calm anxiety, but you can easily meditate at home or even in a quiet place at work.

Different schools of meditation have different rules about how to sit and what to wear but the essentials are simple:

- Sit comfortably in an upright chair in a room where you won't be disturbed, with your feet flat on the ground and your hands in your lap. Close your eyes and imagine a thread is pulling you up from the top of your head – this straightens your spine.
- Breathe slowly and deeply through your nose, imagining the breath travelling down through your lungs and into your stomach and back up again. Make the breaths long by counting to five, or even ten, on the in- and the out-breath.
- Focus on the object of your meditation. This might be simply watching in your mind's eye your breath flowing in and out through your nostrils. Or you could choose a real or imaginary object like a candle or a

flower. Look at it closely, examining its texture and colour. Or focus on a simple word – many people use 'peace' or 'one' or the Eastern sound 'om'.

● Don't worry if your attention wanders – just let the thoughts pass through your mind, watch them go, and bring your concentration gently back to your focus.

Ideally you should do this for 10 to 20 minutes twice a day – set a clock or kitchen-timer so that you don't have to think about time.

The Indian discipline of yoga and the Chinese one of t'ai chi are active forms of meditation that combine breathing techniques with gentle exercise routines in order to restore the energy balance of mind and body. T'ai chi in particular has been described as 'meditation in motion'. Indian and Chinese traditional therapy see ill-health as a sign that the body's vital energy (*prana* in India and *chi* in China) is out of balance (*see* Chapter 6). Both activities have been shown to have beneficial effects on stress-related conditions.

A well-known Western version popular with many office-workers is autogenic training. It has three main positions: the simple sitting, the armchair and the reclining. Each position should be adopted with the eyes shut and the mind told to think only about pleasant and peaceful things.

The training involves 'thinking' your body through six basic exercises in turn to make your neck, shoulders, arms, hands, legs and feet feel heavy and warm, your heartbeat strong and regular, your breathing deep, your stomach relaxed and warm (this also influences breathing) and your forehead cool.

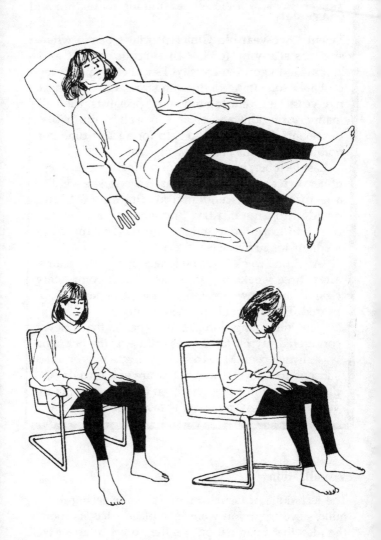

Fig. 4 The three main autogenic positions

Gina's story

Twenty-two-year-old Gina's psoriasis began when she was studying for her final school exams and preparing to go to university. Her doctor said it was probably something to do with stress. Over the next five years she went to numerous specialists, tried all manner of lotions and creams as well as ultraviolet treatments. Sun seemed to help for a short time but nothing solved the problem long term.

Last October, in the midst of setting up a business of her own and with her skin at its worst, she went to a lecture on transcendental meditation (TM) and decided to give it a try. She went on a four-day course to learn the technique and then continued to meditate for 20 minutes twice a day.

'After one week I was no longer using any creams, after three weeks my skin had almost completely cleared, and now even most of the scars have disappeared. That's never happened before.'

'The interesting thing,' says Gina, 'is that I never considered myself to be stressed. I was the one who was always cool. My stress, it seems, has been on a subconscious level. I was not aware of it on a day-to-day basis but my skin had been trying to tell me for years. TM has given me a way to release that stress.'

Visualization

The technique of visualization – literally seeing in your mind's eye what you want take place – has its roots in the idea that imagination has the power to affect well-being and health. The 'will' to live is often talked about but you cannot, for example, *will* your mouth to water, although you can make it water if you *think* about your favourite food.

In the same way many people – both doctors and alternative therapists – believe that the imagination has a tremendous power to activate the body's self-healing abilities. While conventional studies have mostly shown there is no increased effect when visualization is added to meditation, there are many reports of people who have made dramatic recoveries from cancer or horrific injuries by imagining that their disease-fighting white blood cells were white knights on horseback slaying the bad cancer cells, or by visualizing tiny helpers piecing their injured bodies back together again, whole and healthy.

Visualization exercises for people with psoriasis might be to imagine they are lying in the sun, its warmth slowly melting their scaly patches away or walking on a beach with the warm sea breeze blowing the scales away. One sufferer imagined that an invisible 'friend' was gradually eating all the red flakes away, leaving him with silky-smooth and clear skin.

Positive affirmations

Affirmations are positive statements that you repeat over and over in your head several times daily. The most well-known one, suggested by 19th-century French chemist Emile Coué and made famous by Beatle John Lennon, is: 'Every day in every way I am getting better and better'.

Many therapists, however, advise people to be more specific, turning personal negative thoughts or attitudes on their heads. For example, someone with psoriasis might say 'My skin is cool and smooth and clear' or 'My skin is healing by the minute' or 'I am relaxed and at ease with the world'.

It is important always to make it personal – use 'I' and 'my' – and never use negatives; so rather than ' I will not smoke', use 'I have stopped smoking' or 'My lungs are clean and free from smoke'.

Again, this technique relies on the power of the imagination. Practitioners believe that negative thoughts in the subconscious mind have as bad an effect on a person's frame of mind as if spoken out loud. To overcome long-held negative beliefs ('My psoriasis always comes back' or 'I'll never have nice skin') you have to re-programme the subconscious mind. Practitioners say it doesn't matter if you don't actually believe the statement; firstly, because your subconscious mind has to change before you can and, secondly, because just saying something positive, especially if you put real excitement into it, encourages a positive outlook anyway.

Affirmations can also be used to block out that nagging critical voice that often accompanies us as 'background music' day in, day out. You know, the one that says: 'You can't do that', 'Oh, you are stupid', 'You look awful', and so on! Try catching that voice whenever you hear it and immediately and consciously replace the negative thought with a positive one.

Hypnosis/Hypnotherapy

Hypnosis has been given a bad name by stage performers who use the skill to make people bark like dogs and hand over their wallets. But, in the right hands, hypnosis is a powerful medical tool. It is increasingly used by conventional doctors for pain relief, particularly in childbirth, and has been found to be highly effective in relieving stress-related conditions. In one trial, hypnosis was able to ease irritable bowel syndrome, and in another, children on strong chemotherapy drugs vomited less when taught self-hypnosis.

Practitioners believe hypnosis works on two levels. First, when a person is hypnotized the mind falls into a deeply relaxed state which allows all body processes to slow down. This is similar to meditation in that it allows the body to recover from the stresses and strains of daily life. Second, in this state the mind can take on board suggestions that it might reject in normal life. This means that if the practitioner implants ideas that encourage the person to feel more self-confident, more in control and less anxious and stressed, the impact of these suggestions will continue after the person comes out of the trance.

Studies into hypnosis have found that it can relieve stress-related conditions quickly, but there is evidence that this is not so much a result of the power of suggestion as of the deep relaxation which affects the patient's anxiety levels. Many hypnotherapists see themselves more as teachers than healers; they teach their clients the techniques of self-hypnosis (not unlike meditation) so that they can continue the process between visits.

There is very little risk of something unpleasant happening with hypnosis: practitioners say you cannot be hypnotized against your will, or made to do anything you do not really wish to do. But it is important to choose a reputable practitioner.

Psychotherapy

Psychotherapy is another way of trying to reach hidden problems which may be causing stress or emotional distress. The idea is that by pouring out such problems to an understanding and objective stranger, patients not only feel relief but can be helped to deal with whatever is bothering them in a more rational, less anxiety-provoking way.

Practitioners believe that life's rough patches are usually due to:

- *Choice* – where you can't decide which is the right step in a situation and find you are unable to make any move at all.
- *Change* – marriage, divorce, death, retirement and job changes are major life-events, and the strength of feelings they stir up can take you by surprise.
- *Confusion* – feeling distressed but not knowing why, or knowing the reason but not wanting to accept it, or not being able to prevent the problem. An unhappy marriage, emotional abuse, job failure, and anxiety about loved ones can all take their toll if your coping mechanisms are not strong.

There are literally dozens of different types of therapy in this area. For example:

- *Behavioural therapy* believes our behaviour is conditioned by our response to the environment and can be changed with various physical and mental exercises. Often successful with stress-related conditions and irrational fears and phobias.
- *Cognitive therapy* believes previous experiences condition the way we think of ourselves, which in turn affects the way we deal with certain situations. So, for example, a past experience may have made you lack confidence in speaking in public. This therapy would aim to change your thinking to realize that is not the way it always has to be.
- *Gestalt therapy* aims to make people aware of their thoughts and actions by making them conscious of their immediate behaviour, particularly their 'body language'. Often effective for people who are tense or anxious or who have difficulty communicating.
- *Transactional analysis* is based on the theory that inside

everyone there is a child, parent and adult 'self', and through learning about them, people can understand their own behaviour and know when each role is appropriate.

- *Psychodrama* involves groups of people taking turns to act out each other's real-life situations to help learn different ways of dealing with problems. It can release explosive emotions but can be very effective for people who find it difficult to relate to others.

The only sensible way to choose a therapy is to spend some time reading about the different types, pick one that appeals to you, and be prepared to try others if the first doesn't feel right. A personal recommendation can make the choice easier, but therapy is a very individual thing so don't be surprised if what worked for your friend seems like mumbo-jumbo to you.

One-to-one counselling can be expensive and as it tends to go on over several months it is easy to become dependent on your weekly fix. Remember, the idea is to regain your own confidence, not to get answers from the therapist.

Group work

Sometimes group sessions – where people with the same condition can share experiences and vent frustration and fears that might be embarrassing to talk about with non-sufferers – are more helpful than the one-to-one counselling.

People with psoriasis often start to see themselves only in terms of their skin and because of this lose confidence socially. After a period of getting to know each other, a group lets people put aside their skin condition and learn to be themselves again and develop a more reasonable approach to their condition. Some hospitals and psoriasis association branches offer group therapies facilitated by a counsellor.

Creative therapies

Creative therapies include anything that allows people to freely express their bottled-up anger, frustration or grief. They are very helpful in stress-related disorders. Some people find painting or writing can release emotions that have been stored up for years; others find dance, music or drama can provide the outlet.

Aromatherapy

Aromatherapy uses essential oils of aromatic plants to relax the body and stimulate the healing process. How smell actually affects our brain or moods, and ultimately our health, is a bit of a mystery, though it is known that lavender appears to encourage an alpha brainwave pattern (typical of a relaxed state) and jasmine triggers beta rhythms (associated with alertness).

Although serious clinical research into aromatherapy has only recently begun, there have been good results from clinical trials using peppermint oil for irritable bowel disease and tea tree and lavender for wound healing and post-operative stress.

Apart from aiding the relaxation process and controlling the stress which so often exacerbates psoriasis, aromatherapists believe that certain essential oils also boost the immune system.

Oils are usually used diluted in a base oil – such as almond, jojoba or olive oil – for massage, or they can be added to bath water or inhaled in steam. But remember, these are powerful substances, not just perfumes. Except for lavender and tea tree oil, never use them neat; and if you are pregnant, epileptic or suffer from high blood pressure, always consult a qualified clinical aromatherapist first.

The following treatments are useful for psoriasis:

- Wheatgerm oil, mixed with a few drops of benzoin, cajput or bergamot essential oils and applied to affected skin morning and night, soothes irritation and inflammation.
- Lavender oil in the bath reduces inflammation and soothes nervous tension.
- Bergamot acts on anxiety, stress and lack of confidence.
- Sandalwood oil is beneficial for very dry and scaly skin.
- Cedarwood helps the skin and respiratory tract.
- Camomile is anti-inflammatory and soothes stress and aids relaxation.

Flower remedies

Flower remedies or essences are tinctures prepared from wild plants, bushes and trees. They do not treat physical disease but claim to work on a mental and emotional level, helping to stabilize psychological stress factors (such as fear, loneliness, worry, jealousy and insecurity), which practitioners see as the root cause of disease.

Essences have no taste – if anything they may have a vague flavour of the brandy used in small amounts as a preservative – are completely harmless, and work on the same 'imprinting' principle as homoeopathy (*see* page 96). Indeed, conventional doctors say the effect is purely mind over matter because scientific analysis has shown that remedies contain only spring water and alcohol and nothing more.

The most well-known essences are the Bach flower remedies, after the English physician and philosopher

Dr Edward Bach developed his range in the 1920s and 30s. Many other countries have now developed their own range of remedies, based on native wild flowers and more suited, it is held, to the local people.

Remedies suggested for psoriasis often relate to a tense, introverted personality or someone who is ashamed or fearful of rejection. Bach 'Rescue Remedy', a combination remedy which is used in times of crisis to calm physical and mental distress, may be particularly helpful for psoriasis flare-ups at stressful times. But don't wait until the plaques appear – take the remedy immediately you feel stressed. It is also available in a cream.

Flower remedies useful for psoriasis

Bach remedies

Water violet – for a person who prefers to be alone, who seems aloof, proud and reserved, is capable and reliable but will not get personally involved in others' affairs.

Agrimony – for someone who covers up suffering with a cheerful facade, doesn't want to 'be a burden', and often seeks escape through drugs and alcohol.

Crab apple – for someone with feelings of shame and uncleanliness, or fear of contaminating others. Also helps detoxify the system and heal both internal and external wounds.

Willow – for a person who has suffered a misfortune or situation which was felt to be unjust or unfair, and who has become resentful and bitter as a result.

Australian remedies

Billy goat plum – for physical loathing or self-disgust. Brings acceptance of the physical body and sexual pleasure.

Spinifex – heals physically by helping people to understand the emotional issues involved in their condition.

North American remedies

Angelica – offers spiritual protection, strengthens trust and helps to develop strength to face the unknown.

Aloe vera – restores inner balance, helps combat exhaustion and replenish energy for life.

Canadian remedies

Vanilla leaf – encourages affirmation and acceptance of the self. Replaces self-loathing with self-esteem and promotes exuberance, joy and acceptance of self.

CHAPTER 9

Therapies for healing the skin

Other whole-system approaches

So far we have explored the therapies that relate to a suggested cause: food intake, surroundings, and psychological state. But there are also several major natural healing systems that concentrate on treating the whole person rather than just the symptoms which have helped many people relieve or even cure their psoriasis. The most convincing so far are:

- homoeopathy
- acupuncture
- acupressure
- Western herbal medicine
- Chinese herbal medicine
- reflexology

Homoeopathy

Homoeopathy is a complete system of medicine based on principles suggested by Hippocrates in the fifth century BC and developed by a German physician, Dr Samuel Hahnemann, at the start of the 19th century. It is now widely used, particularly in Europe. In Britain, where it has been recognized by an Act of Parliament, homoeopathic medicines are available on the National Health Service, and there are several homoeopathic teaching hospitals. It is said that the Queen never travels anywhere without her box of homoeopathic remedies.

Homoeopathy works on two key principles:

- The 'Principle of Similars' or 'like cures like'.

    In Greek, from which the word 'homoeopathy' comes, *homoios* means 'similar' and *pathos* means 'suffering'. Homoeopaths believe that by giving a minute amount of a substance that would, in a normal dose, cause the symptoms you're trying to cure, the body's own self-healing powers or 'vital force' are jolted into action. For example, that poison most favoured by murder writers, arsenic, is a common homoeopathic remedy for diarrhoea and food poisoning. By contrast, conventional or 'allopathic' medicine generally aims to counteract symptoms by using remedies that are the opposite of the symptom – *allos* meaning 'different' – though it does not always stick to this principle: quinine, for example, which can cause the symptoms of malaria, is also used to cure it.

- The dilution of substances to increase their curative power and prevent unwanted side-effects.

    Homoeopathic remedies are made by steeping plants, minerals and metals in alcohol to create a 'mother tincture'. This is then diluted over and over again with water and shaken vigorously each time, enabling the liquid to retain what practitioners call a 'memory' or 'imprint' of the original substance. Finally the liquid is turned into tiny pills by adding sugar and starch.

Though many homoeopaths are also medical doctors, there is still a good deal of suspicion about the therapy from conventional practitioners who say homoeopathy is a prime example of the 'placebo effect' described on page 76. This is in spite of the fact that research has shown that animals benefit from homoeopathic remedies – and it is hardly likely that they are employing 'mind over matter' techniques.

Homoeopathic remedies have been found to prevent stillbirth in pigs, and other studies in humans and animals have demonstrated that remedies can produce biological changes in hormone levels, enzymes and immune response and pain-killing activity.

Furthermore, homoeopathy has come successfully through the most rigorous scientific tests demanded by doctors themselves – the 'double-blind' trial, where neither the patients treated nor the testers know whether the remedy is real or fake. In a recent such study in Britain on 50 people, those receiving the real remedy were significantly better after three months, while patients taking the fake remedy had deteriorated.

Another objection to homoeopathic remedies is that they are so watered down they may contain no molecules of the original substance at all. Though there is as yet no scientifically acceptable reason for how a remedy with no measurably active ingredient can possibly work, the flip side of this argument is that precisely because they are so dilute, homoeopathic remedies are extremely safe, even for babies and small children.

Because homoeopathy treats people rather than diseases, there are no blanket remedies for particular conditions. Each person is treated individually. Initially you can try to treat yourself or your family – remedies are available in most healthfood shops and many pharmacies (*see* page 101 for suggestions for common skin conditions) – but with complex conditions such as psoriasis, you will probably need the help of a trained homoeopath.

The first consultation with a homoeopath usually takes an hour to an hour and a half. Practitioners have upwards of 2,500 remedies to choose from and base their prescription on their assessment of your personality, state of mind, reactions and lifestyle, as well as your medical history and symptoms. Normally you will be given one dose, then another about half an hour later. Unlike conventional medicines, homoeopathic remedies do not need to be taken over a period of time: if the right remedy is chosen, one dose may be enough.

However, with complex conditions like psoriasis – which homoeopaths believe indicates imbalances in the harmony of the body – the first remedy may 'decide' to address an underlying problem rather than act immediately on the symptoms. Your skin condition, for example, could be related to suppressed grief, a lack of self confidence, or a weakened liver.

There may be several hidden problems and several remedies may be needed before the actual symptoms disappear, although it is likely that you will start to feel better in yourself, even if your skin does not immediately improve. How long the cure takes also depends on how long the underlying problems have been suppressed.

Your practitioner will probably want to see you about two weeks after the first treatment to ensure that the condition is, literally, moving in the right direction. Homoeopaths believe that disease moves down the body and out through the feet or fingers. So if the root cause is being addressed, your skin should gradually clear, starting from the centre and upper part of your body. If this is not happening and you are feeling depressed, the remedy given was not the correct one for your case.

Some homoeopaths also believe their remedies are able to break the genetic links of diseases like psoriasis and stop it passing on to other generations, but there is as yet no proof of this and critics are highly sceptical.

Generally, homoeopathic and conventional treatments can be carried out side by side. Homoeopaths, though, believe steroid creams reduce the body's own healing powers and may make their remedies less effective. Nevertheless, it is important not to give up steroids without consulting a medically-trained practitioner because a sudden stop can be harmful.

John's story

John had a high-powered, high-pressure job when his psoriasis started. When he finally tried homoeopathy he had changed to something more low key, and for most of the time had just a few small dry red patches on his skin. But whenever his confidence was threatened or there was a stressful situation, he felt unable to cope and within a short time his skin became red and sore, then extra dry and scaly. He also craved salt.

The homoeopath talked to him for a long time about his life. He revealed that he felt his parents had always expected a lot of him and he was always worried that he would make mistakes in life. He had realized that the stress in his high-powered job was not good for his health but even after changing his job, he still had rushes of inadequacy. These were compounded by the fact that he felt condemned by his parents for 'giving up' and doing an ordinary job. The homoeopath prescribed *natrum mur* (based on sodium) to build self-esteem, and other remedies which focused on dryness.

Over the next three months, which was the start of winter when his skin was generally worse, John had no flare-ups and the usual marks on his skin faded.

Common homoeopathic remedies for psoriasis

Although no two people would necessarily be given the same homoeopathic treatment for psoriasis, some commonly used remedies are:

- *arsen alb* – for very dry, rough, scaly skin which gets worse in the cold; or for when there are small red pimples covered in scurf, which burn and itch (often accompanied by feelings of anxiety and restlessness)
- *graphites* – for dry and cracked skin which itches and bleeds (can also be used if the psoriasis patches become infected and ooze a sticky discharge)
- *sulphur* – for dry and burning skin with a crawling itch all over the body (scratching gives temporary relief but is followed by burning pain and soreness; the sufferer cannot tolerate heat or cold)
- *sepia* – for skin which feels itchy and raw; patches have yellow-brown cracks but stay dry with no discharge

---

Acupuncture

Acupuncture has been used in China for more than 5,000 years. It is based on the belief in an energy or life-force that flows not only through the human body but also throughout the universe. This force – called *qi* or *chi* (pronounced 'chee') in China, *ki* in Japan, and *prana* in India – is a balance of two opposing energies known as *yin* and *yang*. It flows along 12 main *meridians* or channels which cover the entire body. If the flow becomes blocked or unbalanced – by inherited sensitivities, bad diet, strong emotions, drugs, infections, climate, too little or too much work, exercise or sex – the result is ill-health and disease.

Acupuncturists insert super-fine stainless steel, silver or gold needles into any of 2,000 pressure points on the meridians to restore the balance of the energy and thus the body's well-being. They may also use a technique called *moxibustion*, which involves placing a smoulder-ing herb (mugwort) on the needle or twirling it nearby to clear the channel and encourage the flow of energy through the body.

Before treating you, an acupuncturist will follow the four methods of Chinese diagnosis: observing, listening and smelling, interrogating, pulse-taking and palpation. They will ask you about your past and present health and lifestyle; observe your posture, the way you walk and sit; study your tongue, your hair, your skin tone; lis-ten to your voice – is it whiney (dysfunctional lung ener-gy) or sharp (possible problems with liver energy)?; feel your abdomen; and test the tempo of the pulses of each of the 12 meridians.

The needles are generally inserted to a depth of about 5 millimetres (a quarter of an inch) and left in for five to 30 minutes. The sensation should not be painful, though you may feel a slight ache or tingle where the needles are. Some practitioners use an electrified probe to pass a weak electric current either down the needles or directly onto the skin without breaking the surface.

Because of the possibility of infection from misused needles, it is important to ensure you visit a qualified and accredited acupuncturist who follows strict steriliza-tion procedures (*see* Chapter 10 for how to check creden-tials and *Appendix A* for addresses of reputable organizations).

No one has yet come up with scientific evidence to prove the existence of the meridian system, but numer-ous studies both in China and the West have shown that acupuncture works well in many circumstances. The once very sceptical medical profession is increasingly advising patients for whom conventional medicine has failed to give acupuncture a try.

Many hospitals now use acupuncture as a pain reliever. It is often used in childbirth, even for caesarian operations, because it allows women to remain conscious and forgo drugs that may affect the baby.

Research shows that acupuncture encourages the body to release natural pain-killing hormones called *endorphins* and *enkephalins* into the nervous system. Another suggestion is that the nerves carrying pressure messages brought on by the needle or by massaging the acupuncture point reach the brain faster than those carrying pain messages. This causes the brain to close the 'gate' to later messages because it can only deal with so many at once.

Acupuncturists and Chinese herbalists (*see* page 113) believe skin conditions are evidence of disharmony in the lungs, and the well-being of the lungs reflects the extent to which people make healthy, constructive connections with the world they live in. Bad lungs suggest an alienated person. So therapy is often aimed at strengthening the flow of chi between the lungs and the skin.

Though there has been little research into the effect of acupuncture on chronic diseases in the West, Chinese research has demonstrated success with a variety of disorders, including psoriatic arthritis, high blood pressure, depression, intestinal disorders, asthma, eczema, hay fever and migraine.

However, some medically-trained acupuncturists in Britain (using hour-long treatments, once a week at first, then every two weeks, over a period of three to four months) have reported surprising and lasting success with 70 per cent of psoriasis sufferers (*see* case studies box on page 105). They suggest that acupuncture affects the release of *serotonin*, a drug which plays a role in controlling depression and stress and dilates the blood vessels in the skin, improving circulation.

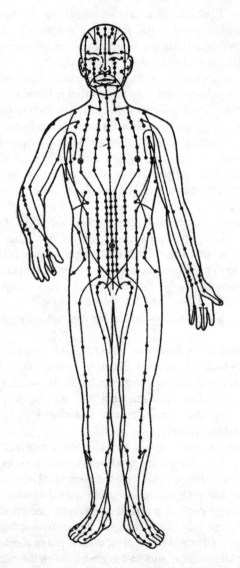

Fig. 5 The meridian system in Chinese acupuncture

Case studies

- Eighteen-year-old Jenny had suffered from guttate psoriasis for ten years. She had her first acupuncture treatment just after being discharged from hospital for the umpteenth time. After three sessions in a month, her skin improved; and after a total of 20 sessions over the next nine months her skin was virtually clear. The following year she had a minor flare-up which was treated with a single session. Four years later, her skin remains virtually clear.

- Thirty-nine-year-old Stephanie suffered from psoriasis for 14 years and was particularly disturbed by the itching. She had tried steroid creams without lasting effect. After her first acupuncture treatment the itching subsided but returned to the same level two days later. After the second treatment a week later, the itching again subsided and rose, but less dramatically. After the third treatment, it dropped away completely and did not rise again for several months.

- Jackson, 66, had psoriasis for 40 years. After a total of 16 treatment sessions, his skin was almost clear, and has remained so with three-monthly 'top-up' treatments.

Acupressure

Acupressure is essentially acupuncture without needles. Practitioners use their fingers and hands to apply pressure to points on the meridians to stimulate and restore the flow of the life-force to areas where it is depleted. The sensation is of a firm massage, although when the right point is found it can feel quite painful at first.

You can practise basic acupressure techniques yourself. With clean, warm, dry hands, hold your palm briefly over an acupressure point. Then move the tip of your finger until you feel a slight dip and press lightly until you feel the muscle relax. Increase the pressure slowly until the point feels neither warm nor cold, and pulses slightly. This usually takes about three minutes. Then ease off gently and move to the next point.

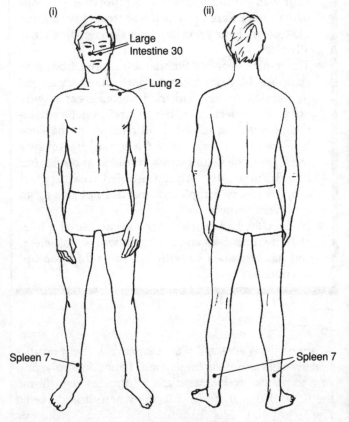

Fig. 6 Acupressure points for psoriasis

(iii)

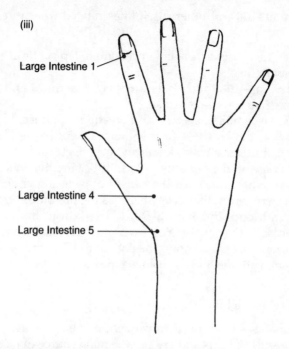

Large Intestine 1

Large Intestine 4

Large Intestine 5

Acupressure points for psoriasis

Press at least two of these points each day.

- *Large intestine Pt 1* – just below the right-hand corner of the nail on the forefinger
- *Large intestine Pt 4* – on the palm in the centre of the muscle below the thumb, and on the upper side of the hand in the muscle between the thumb and forefinger
- *Large intestine Pt 5* – on the upper side of the wrist at the base of the thumb
- *Large intestine Pt 30* – in the crease of the nostrils
- *Spleen Pt 7* – at the back of the leg at the base of the calf muscle
- *Lung 2* – in the dip just below the shoulder-end of the collarbone

There are several other disciplines related to acupressure:

- *Shen Tao* – uses a very light pressure to tap subtle energy patterns.
- *Jin Shen* – the touch lasts for several minutes and is more like a massage stroke.
- *Do-In* – combines exercise and breathing routines.
- *Shiatsu*, the Japanese form – the practitioner uses fingers, thumbs, elbows, knees and even feet to add extra leverage on the pressure points. In Britain, the Shiatsu Society has translated the benefit of restoring chi into Western terms: the society believes the pressure stimulates blood and lymph fluid circulation, helps to release toxins and tension from muscles, and balances hormones. It also allows the patient to relax and get in touch with the body's healing abilities.

Herbal medicine

Plants have been used to prevent or heal disease for thousands of years and are still the main source of medicine for four out of five people in the world. Some plants have also provided the raw materials for today's modern drugs. For example, the heart drug *digoxin* comes from foxgloves, *alkaloids* used to treat leukaemia and Hodgkin's lymphoma are extracted from the Madagascan periwinkle, the active ingredient in *aspirin* comes from willow bark, the herb *curare* used in South American Indian blowpipes contains an agent now used by surgeons to relax a patient's muscles before an operation, and *diosgenin* from Mexican wild yam is the base of many steroid preparations.

All these drugs have been produced by isolating one part of the natural substance and reproducing it synthetically. The pharmaceutical industry argues that these copy chemicals are more consistent and can therefore be given in more accurate doses, unlike plants that can vary from season to season. But herbalists say synthetic drugs contain only the active ingredient, leaving out many others that make up the whole plant.

This 'whole plant' combination may relieve several symptoms that occur together, not just the most obvious one, and may also counteract any nasty side-effects of the active ingredient. For example, herbalists use the plant *Ephedra* to treat asthma. A side-effect of its active ingredient, *ephedrine*, is raised blood pressure, but the other constituents of the plant (taken in a herbal prescription but excluded from synthetic drugs) counter this side-effect and maintain normal blood pressure.

Meadowsweet, the herbal equivalent of aspirin, also illustrates this point. Like aspirin, it contains salicylic acid which can cause stomach ulcers if taken alone or too frequently. But as meadowsweet also contains tannin and mucilage, natural protectors and healers of the stomach lining, the effect of the acid is balanced.

Doctors are frequently sceptical of herbal medicines because they know little about them (except those they have tested by '20th-century standards') and because no one remedy suits everyone with a particular condition. And while research is being done in various ways in the Far East, particularly China, the findings are often not taken seriously by conventional Western medicine. Nevertheless, there is little doubt that many people do benefit greatly from herbal medicine.

Herbalists usually view psoriasis as an *auto-immune* disease: that is, one where the body's defences have for some reason turned against its own tissues. The remedies most often used seek to reduce toxins wherever they are accumulating in the body, and pay particular attention to the health of the liver. Practitioners see symptoms as the body's way of trying to restore internal

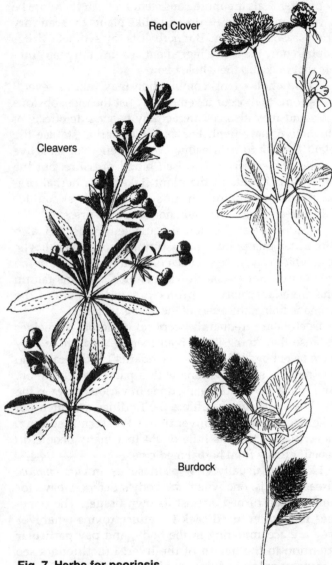

Fig. 7 Herbs for psoriasis

Red Clover

Cleavers

Burdock

Herbs that may help psoriasis

- *Red clover and sarsaparilla* – key herbs in psoriasis and eczema; used to detoxify the system, cleanse the blood and encourage good use of nutrients in food. Sarsaparilla is also used to control chronic arthritis.
- *Burdock* – one of the best herbal remedies for dry scaly skin. Make a tea by simmering one teaspoonful of burdock root in a cup of water for 15 minutes. It can also be combined with yellow dock root, red clover and sarsaparilla and taken three times a day for up to three months.
- *Elder* – a hot infusion of elderflowers stimulates the circulation, causes sweating and cleanses the system of toxins. Ointments containing the root and bark of elder soothe plaques.
- *Dock* – a liver tonic with a high iron content and an aid to weak digestion (both possible causes of psoriasis). Dock is also a good detoxifier and stimulates congested blood and lymph fluids. Take as a tincture or tea, or use as a lotion to counter inflammation.
- *Watercress* – a blood cleanser that livens up the digestion, improves absorption of food and increases circulation. It stimulates the liver and helps detoxify the system as well as pepping up the immune system. Also good as a stress tonic because of its large number of vitamins, mineral and trace elements.
- *Cleavers* – as a lotion is a treatment against psoriasis, eczema and other skin conditions. Taken as a tea it cleanses the lymphatic system and reduces glandular swelling.

The Celtic concoction

In the green heart of the Republic of Ireland, a clinic is promoting a therapy for psoriasis that has been handed down and used with success by four generations of the Walsh family, traditional Irish herbalists.

The Cherryfields Clinic's 'Celtic concoction' consists of almost 30 traditional Irish plants used in a three-stage therapy. Patients first apply a cream, containing ten herbs gathered from many different parts of the island, six times a day for up to four months. This is to reduce the scaling and bring the skin into a condition as close to normal as possible. Although tedious, the cream is not unpleasant to use.

Along with this, the patient takes a detoxifying medicine made of six herbs to attack the roots of the problem, which the Walshes believe results from a hormonal imbalance. Next comes a hormone tincture medication made from 14 plants. This is taken for up to nine months and seeks to rebalance the hormonal systems and nudge the body into a position where it can again look after itself. In addition, patients are advised to stay away from acid food, alcohol and smoking.

From his observations of this treatment over the past ten years, therapist John Woulfe believes that over 50 per cent of patients who have stuck rigorously to the regime have cleared their skin, without recurrences, within a year. A further group who were not able to stick to the schedule so closely, did eventually become clear.

It is not a cheap treatment, costing up to £200 a month initially and dropping to about £100 a month at the tincture stage, but its reputation does pull people to the clinic from all over Europe as well as North America.

balance, so although they may give you a lotion to ease the immediate symptoms, they may also prescribe remedies which aim to deal with the root cause (liver overload, for example) and stimulate the body's own healing powers. And they will usually give advice on diet and exercise to promote overall good health.

Herbal remedies come in many forms. They may be eaten directly (cooked or uncooked); given as teas or infusions; added to bathwater; inhaled; or made into tablets, creams, ointments, poultices or highly-concentrated liquids called tinctures or decoctions. Some are fast acting, others are gentle treatments which take time to work.

You can grow your own plants, buy them living or dried, or visit a trained herbalist. There are any number of good books available on preparing and using herbal medicine – but remember, herbs can be as potent and poisonous as drugs. Treat them with respect, do not exceed the prescribed doses, and never use herbal medicine during pregnancy without professional advice.

Chinese herbal medicine

Chinese herbal medicine, like acupuncture, is part of the system of traditional Chinese medicine and is based on the principle of balancing body energy or *chi*. Unlike Western practitioners who generally use only plants or herbs, Chinese herbalists also draw on a sometimes unnerving but frequently effective collection of plants, fungi, wood and, occasionally, animal parts.

Recent research has shown this form of medicine to be very effective in treating certain types of eczema, and trials are under way to investigate the benefits for other conditions, including psoriasis, asthma, migraine and irritable bowel syndrome.

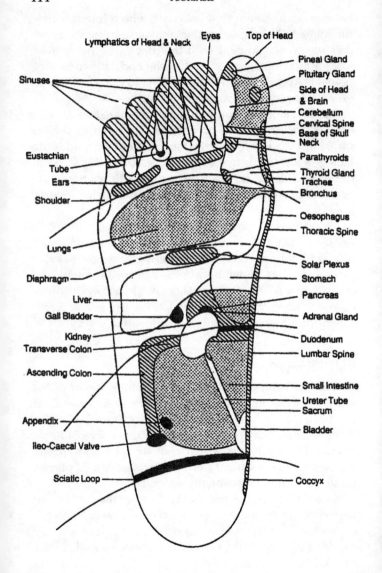

Fig. 8 Reflex zones on the right foot

However, some of the herbs are very toxic and have the potential to cause serious damage to the digestive system if used carelessly or inappropriately. In Britain, over 70 women who took a slimming treatment (unheard of in Chinese medicine) containing Chinese herbs are now suffering from severe kidney damage. In other instances patients treating themselves have not fully realized the potency of their 'brew' of herbs and have suffered liver problems. Of course, side-effects can occur with the misuse of any medicine, but this is less likely to happen if you use a qualified practitioner.

Reflexology

Reflexologists believe every part of the body is linked to points or zones on the feet by the same sort of energy lines used in acupuncture and acupressure. They, too, believe that illness is caused by blockages and imbalances in these lines. By massaging the correct point on the feet reflexologists can clear the channels and get the natural healing powers working again. The practice dates back to ancient Egypt (perhaps earlier) and is claimed to promote both healing and relaxation.

Focus points for psoriasis are those which affect the liver, kidneys and lungs; but massage to the areas which affect the solar plexus and diaphragm (particularly related to stress) may also prove beneficial. Vacuflex, a modern version of reflexology that uses felt boots and silicon pads to apply controlled pressure, is said to be particularly effective for psoriasis.

CHAPTER 10

How to find and choose a practitioner

Tips and guidelines for seeking out reliable help

Natural forms of medicine have enjoyed a boom in popularity in most Western countries over recent years, but it is still not always easy to find the right therapist. Once you've decided which therapy to try, there is no real system (like the conventional medicine routine of referrals) to point you in the right direction. This means that you need to take much more responsibility yourself, both for tracking down a suitable therapist and for checking that he or she is experienced and good at the job.

Finding a good practitioner, whatever the discipline, is often a matter of tuning in to the 'bush telegraph'. A personal recommendation from someone you know is a good place to start, and is even better if it claims success with the same condition as yours. If you belong to a patient support group, you will almost certainly find other members who have tried natural techniques of one sort or another.

A word of warning though – just because a particular therapy cleared your friend's lesions, there is no guarantee that it will clear yours. As you will know from this book, individualism is important in natural medicine and lack of success does not necessarily mean either the therapy or the therapist is no good.

If you don't know anyone with personal experience,

then ask around relations, friends, neighbours and work-mates. If you still draw a blank, try your family doctor's clinic. Not all doctors – or their staff – will respond help-fully, and if all you get is dire warnings, ignore them. But increasingly, medical practitioners are broadminded about such requests. Many may have their own interests in particular areas of natural medicine and may even be trained therapists themselves. In Britain, for example, nearly 40 per cent of doctors have some training in unconventional approaches such as homoeopathy and acupuncture and some clinics now have natural thera-pists working on the premises. (In some countries certain consultations are paid for by the state health service.)

Even clinics unfamiliar with alternative medicine may be aware of natural therapists practising in the area – if only because patients will have told them about success-ful treatments – and they may be prepared to give you the names of the most popular ones, even if they cannot recommend a specific one. Larger towns often have a natural health centre staffed by practitioners from a vari-ety of disciplines. As therapists usually know one anoth-er, the centre may be able to point you in the right direction if the type of therapy you want is not on offer.

Other local sources include libraries and healthfood shops: the names of successful therapists are usually well known. Again, if you get a recommendation for another type of therapy, try asking that therapist if he or she knows of someone practising the therapy you have in mind.

National organizations representing particular natur-al medicine disciplines, or 'umbrella' organizations rep-resenting a range of therapies, may be able to supply you with a list of registered and approved practitioners, as well as general information about the discipline. The national or local psoriasis society or association may also be able to advise you (*see Appendix A*).

Selecting a therapist

If you are lucky you'll find a therapist you feel comfortable with through direct personal recommendation. But
if this doesn't happen and you have to do more research,
there are certain things you need to bear in mind as you
sift through the possibilities.

While most therapists are well-trained, caring and
competent people, it is not difficult in some countries for
those who are not so reliable to set themselves up in
practice. This is particularly true in Britain, where there
are almost no restrictions on who may practise what in
the field of natural therapies. In response to this situation, a British Medical Association report on natural
medicine published in 1993 recommended that anyone
considering attending a non-conventional therapist
should ask the following questions:

- What are the therapist's training and qualifications?
- How long has the therapist been in practice?
- Does the therapist belong to a recognized professional
  body which is governed by a code of conduct?
- Does the therapist have professional indemnity insur-
  ance?

Don't be afraid to ask such questions when booking an
appointment. Anyone worth seeing will expect your
questions and you should steer clear of anyone who
sounds vague or shifty about answering. It also pays to
be wary of being treated by anyone, including a medical
doctor, who has done only a weekend course in the therapy on offer.

Checking professional organizations

If a therapist belongs to a professional organization, it is
a good idea to get more information about the organization itself. Some groups genuinely keep a check on their

members, while others seem interested only in collecting membership fees and manufacturing credibility. Questions to ask include:

- When was it founded? If it's new, don't reject it out of hand – ask why it was formed.
- How many members does it have?
- Does it have members nationwide? Groups which have been going for 50 years and have plenty of members may be better organized and supportive than those started last week in someone's living room. On the other hand, a new group may be more innovative, know all the up-to-date research, and be more enthusiastic.
- Is it part of a larger network of professional organizations? Bodies representing the major therapies often belong to an umbrella organization which promotes the aims and standards of natural medicine in general. Groups that 'do their own thing' entirely may be less likely to adhere to recognized professional and ethical standards.
- Does it accept only members with recognized qualifications? If so, what are those qualifications (see below for questions to ask)? Large professional bodies may be linked with colleges which train therapists or set standards to oversee training. However, beware of organizations whose executives are closely allied with one particular school or college – their assessment of qualifications may not be independent.
- Does it have a code of ethics, a schedule of standards, a complaints mechanism and disciplinary procedures for members who fail in the standards?
- Is it a charity, educational trust or private company? Charities should promote the therapy and service the interests of the public in a non-profitmaking way. Private companies are generally more interested in financial rewards.

● Are members covered by a professional indemnity
  insurance against accident and malpractice? This is an
  important safeguard and points to an overall profes-
  sionalism and concern for patient welfare.

Checking training and qualifications

Next, you may want more details about the therapist's
qualifications. Do the letters after their name just mean
they belong to an organization, or do they indicate in-
depth study? Information from the therapist's organization may explain this and what the recognized
qualification is, or the therapist may have a patients'
information leaflet. If neither of these is available, you
need to ask:

● How long is the training?
● Is the training full or part time? If it is part time, is the
  overall training time equal to a full-time course or is it
  a short-cut ?
● Does the training include seeing patients under supervision? Qualifications which are purely theoretical do
  not tell you much about someone's ability to treat people, and make it less likely that the therapist has had a
  substantial training.
● Is the qualification recognized? If so, by whom? The
  really important thing you need to know is whether
  the qualification is recognized by an independent
  authority, not just the school or college which supplied
  the training.

Making the choice

Once you know all you can about the therapist's background, making a final choice really comes down to
intuition and trying them out. The luxuriousness of the

premises may suggest that someone is popular and financially successful, but it doesn't necessarily tell you that the therapist is good. But if the surroundings feel 'wrong' or the therapist or practice staff make you feel uncomfortable, then be guided by your feelings – don't be afraid to cancel appointments, or even leave, if you do not feel happy with the person, the place or the treatment.

Precautions

If you need to undress for the therapy, feel free to ask for someone you trust to be present if this would make you feel more comfortable. If the therapist refuses to allow someone else to be present, leave. It goes without saying that any sexual advances made by a therapist are unethical, but if anything makes you uneasy on that score, leave at once. If a therapist wishes to touch you on your breasts or genitals, your permission should be sought first.

Do not stop any conventional drug treatments suddenly without first discussing it with your family doctor. Be wary if you are not asked what medications you are taking, and especially wary of a therapist who tells you to stop taking any medication prescribed by your doctor. Responsible therapists and family doctors should be happy to discuss you and your medication with each other.

Query any suggestion that you pay for treatment in advance. Obviously with busy clinics you may need to book sessions in advance, and a therapist may suggest a certain number of sessions will be needed, but you should be able to cancel sessions that prove unnecessary, without penalty, provided you give adequate notice (usually 24 hours). Just occasionally a therapist may ask for advance payment for special tests or medicines, but check carefully exactly what payment is for and obtain a detailed receipt.

Beware of anyone who 'guarantees' you a cure. There is no such thing.

What to do if things go wrong

The most common reason why people feel dissatisfied with a therapist is that the treatment has not made them better. If this happens the first thing to ask yourself is whether you gave it a fair trial. Did you go into it with a positive outlook? Did you follow all the recommendations? Did you keep going for long enough? Many natural therapies need time to work and some may even make you feel worse before you get better.

Next, do you feel the therapist was genuinely trying to help? No therapy – conventional or unconventional – can guarantee success. Remember, too, that psoriasis is a complex individual condition and therapies work at an individual level, so the one that works for your friend may not work for you.

However, if you feel the therapist is incompetent, that he or she caused you harm, took risks or acted unprofessionally or unethically (whether the treatment was successful or not), you should do something about it, if for no other reason than to protect future patients.

Discuss your concerns with the therapist if you feel you can – he or she may be unaware of the problem and only too ready to put it right once it is pointed out. If the therapist works in a centre or clinic, you may feel it is better to tell the management, who have a duty to treat complaints seriously and discreetly.

If this does not solve the problem, report the practitioner to the relevant professional body. This is why it is important to choose a practitioner who is a member of a body with a code of conduct (although, in Britain at least, most of these bodies have little regulatory power and cannot stop someone practising, although they may expel the therapist from their organization).

Voice your concerns to whoever recommended you to the therapist – and anyone else who may be affected. Ultimately bad publicity can be the most effective sanction. But be careful here: think through your complaint carefully and try all other approaches first. Making allegations without good reason may land you in court.

If you believe you are entitled to compensation, you will need the help of a lawyer or consumers' or citizens' rights association for advice on suing the therapist – but be prepared for this to be expensive. If a criminal action is involved, go to the police first.

Conclusion

Despite the occasional scare story, most natural therapists are caring, reputable professionals who have invested much time and money in their training and who put great effort into their practice. Many spend just as long training as conventional doctors, and are equally dedicated, though often not so well paid.

There is an onus on you as the patient to choose carefully and find out as much about the therapy as you can beforehand. But this is no bad thing. Taking responsibility for your own health, searching out the right therapist and being actively involved in treatment can be an important part of the healing process.

Of course, in the end it is also up to you to decide whether the treatment is helping and whether you should continue. If it isn't helpful, do not give up hope – a different approach may work wonders. In psoriasis there is no categorical right answer which is the same for every person. Trying natural therapies broadens the options and increases the possibilities of success.

Useful organizations

The following listing of organizations is for information only and does not imply any endorsement, nor do the organizations listed necessarily agree with the views expressed in this book.

PSORIASIS ASSOCIATIONS

AUSTRALASIA

Auckland Psoriasis Society
PO Box 3062
Auckland 1
New Zealand

Psoriasis Association of New South Wales
c/o Skin and Cancer Foundation
376 Victoria Street
Darlinghurst
NSW 2010, Australia

MIDDLE EAST

Psoriasis Association of Israel
PO Box 13275
Tel Aviv
Israel
Tel 866 545

NORTH AMERICA

Canadian Psoriasis Foundation
PO Box 5036
Armdale
Halifax
Nova Scotia B3L 4M6, Canada

National Psoriasis Foundation
6415 SW Canyon Court, Suite 200
Portland
Oregon 97221, USA

Psoriasis Research Institute
600 Town and Country Village
Palo Alto
California 94070, USA

SOUTHERN AFRICA

South African Psoriasis Association
c/o 166 Herbert Baker Street
Groenkloof
Pretoria 0181
South Africa

UK AND EIRE

**Psoriasis Association in Great
Britain and Ireland**
7 Milton Street
Northampton
Northamptonshire NN2 7JG, UK
Tel 01604 711129

NATURAL MEDICINE
ORGANIZATIONS

INTERNATIONAL

**International Federation of
Practitioners of Natural
Therapeutics**
46 Pulens Crescent
Sheet
Petersfield
Hampshire GU31 4DH, UK
Tel 01730 266 790
Fax 01730 260 058

AUSTRALASIA

**Australian Natural Therapies
Association**
PO Box 308
Melrose Park
South Australia 5039
Tel 8 297 9533
Fax 8 297 0003

**Australian Traditional Medicine
Society**
Suite 3, First floor
120 Blaxland Road
Ryde
New South Wales 2112, Australia
Tel 2 808 2825
Fax 2 809 7570

**New Zealand Natural Health
Practitioners Accreditation
Board**
PO Box 37-491
Auckland
New Zealand
Tel 9 625 9966

NORTH AMERICA

**American Association of
Naturopathic Physicians**
2800 East Madison Street
Suite 200
Seattle
Washington 98112, USA
Tel 206 323 7610
Fax 206 323 7612

**American Holistic Medical
Association**
6728 Old McLean Village Drive
McLean, VA 22101, USA
Tel 703 556 9222

**Canadian Holistic Medicine
Association**
700 Bay Street
PO Box 101, Suite 604
Toronto
Ontario M5G 1Z6, Canada
Tel 416 599 0447

UK AND EIRE

Aromatherapy Organisations Council
3 Latymer Close
Braybooke
Market Harborough
Leicester LE16 8LN
Tel/fax 01858 434242

British Acupuncture Council
Park House, Suite D
206-208 Latimer Road
London W10 6RE
Tel 0181 964 0222
Fax 0181 964 0333
Registers practitioners in both acupuncture and traditional Chinese herbal medicine.

British Association for Counselling
1 Regent Place
Rugby
Warwickshire CV21 2PJ
Tel 01788 578328/9

British Complementary Medicine Association
39 Prestbury Road
Pitville
Cheltenham
Gloucestershire GL52 2PT
Tel 01242 226770
Fax 01242 226778
Umbrella organization representing organizations outside CCAM (see page 128)

British Holistic Medical Association
Trust House
Royal Shrewsbury Hospital South
Shrewsbury
Shropshire SY3 8XF
Tel 01743 261155
Fax 01743 353637
Association of medical professionals working for changes in attitudes and approaches in the National Health Service.

British Homoeopathic Association
27 Devonshire Street
London W1N 1RJ
Tel 0171 935 2163
Members are medically trained practitioners. Send stamped addressed envelope for information and list of members.

British Medical Acupuncture Society
Newton House
Newton Lance
Lower Whitley
Warrington
Cheshire WA4 4JA
Tel 01925 730 727
Members are medical doctors and dentists who have trained in acupuncture.

British Society for Allergy and Environmental Medicine
Acorns
Romsey Road
Cadnam
Southampton
Hampshire SO4 2NN
Write for information on clinical ecology and environmental medicine.

British Society of Experimental and Clinical Hypnosis
c/o Dr Michael Heap
University of Sheffield Centre for Psychotherapeutic Studies
16 Claremont Crescent
Sheffield
South Yorkshire S10 2TA
Tel 0114 824 970

British Society of Medical and Dental Hypnosis
National Office
17 Keppelview Road
Kimberworth
Rotherham
Lancashire SG1 2AR
Tel 01709 554 558

Cherryfields Clinic
Cherryfields House
Ballysimon Road
Limerick
Republic of Ireland
Tel 353 6141 5588
Specializes in traditional Celtic herbal remedies. Also found at the Hale Clinic (see below).

Council for Complementary and Alternative Medicine (CCAM)
Park House, Suite D
206-208 Latimer Road
London W10 6RE
Tel 0181 968 3862
Fax 0181 968 3469

Institute for Complementary Medicine
PO Box 194
London SE16 1QZ
Tel 0171 237 5165
Fax 0171 237 5175

Just Natural Dead Sea Health and Beauty Spa
Unit G2 The Seabed Centre
Wyncolls Road
Severalls Park
Colchester
Essex CO4 4HT
Tel 01206 752852

National Institute of Medical Herbalists
9 Palace Gate
Exeter
Devon EX1 1JA

Natural Medicines Society
Edith Lewis House
Ilkeston
Derbyshire DE7 8EJ

Research Council for Complementary Medicine
60 Great Ormond Street
London WC1N 3JF
Tel 0171 833 8897
Fax 0171 278 7412

Society for the Promotion of Nutritional Therapy
PO Box 47
Heathfield
East Sussex TN21 8ZX
Tel 01435 867 007
Fax 01435 868 033

Society of Homoeopaths
2 Artizan Road
Northampton
Northamptonshire NN1 4HU
Tel 01604 21400
Registers non-medically qualified homoeopaths who have completed a four-year training course followed by one year clinical supervision. Send stamped addressed envelope for list of members.

The Alternative Centre
The White House
Roxby Place
Fulham
London SW6 1RS
Tel 0171 381 2298
Specialist holistic health centre for psoriasis sufferers.

The Hale Clinic
7 Park Crescent
London W1
Tel 0171 631 0156
Offers a range of therapies plus a comprehensive library and natural medicine shop.

UK Council for Psychotherapy
Regent's College
Inner Circle
Regent's Park
London NW1 4NS
Tel 0171 487 7554

Useful further reading

Acupressure Techniques, Julian Kenyon (Thorsons, UK, 1987)

The Alternative Health Guide, Brian Inglis and Ruth West (Michael Joseph, UK, 1984)

Beat Psoriasis, Sandra Gibbons (Thorsons, UK, 1992)

Better Health Through Natural Healing, Ross Tratler (McGraw-Hill, USA, 1987)

The Complete Relaxation Book, James Hewitt (Rider, UK, 1987)

Diets to Help Psoriasis, Harry Clements (Thorsons, UK, 1981)

The Greening of Medicine, Patrick Pietroni (Gollancz, UK, 1990)

The Guide to Bach Flower Remedies, Julian Barnard (C W Daniel, UK, 1979)

Guide to Complementary Medicine and Therapies, Anne Woodham (Health Education Authority, UK, 1994)

Nutritional Medicine, Stephen Davies and Alan Stewart (Pan Books, UK, 1987)

The Reader's Digest Family Guide to Alternative Medicine, ed. Patrick Pietroni (Reader's Digest Association, UK/USA, 1991)

The Rowland Remedy, John Rowland (Javelin Books, UK, 1986)

Teach Yourself Meditation, James Hewitt (Hodder and Stoughton, UK, 1978)

Index

acupressure 96, 105–108
acupuncture 50, 54, 55, 96, 101–105
additives 27, 56, 67
affirmations 25, 87–88
agrimony 94
alcohol 34, 45, 56, 58, 61
allergen test 68
allergies 5, 9, 11, 20, 21, 25, 26, 30–31, 50, 57, 59–60, 65, 67, 70
aloe vera 27, 95
alpha brainwave 92
Anatolia, Turkey 74
angelica 95
animal fats 20, 57, 58
antipuritics 28
apocrine glands 6
arachidonic acid 20, 62
aromatherapy 28, 92–93
arsen alb 101
arthritis 14–15, 71
Australian flower remedies 94
Austrian peat moor bath 75
autogenic training 84–85
auto-immune disorders 17, 109

Bach, Dr Edward 94
Bach flower remedies 81, 93–95
bacteria 9, 17, 22, 56, 57
baths 27–29, 39
behavioural therapy 90
bergamot 93
billy goat plum 94

Blue Lagoon, Iceland 74
bromine 70
burdock 111

calcipotriol 39, 41, 42
camomile 75, 93
Canadian flower remedies 95
candidiasis 57
capillaries 6, 9
cedarwood 93
Celtic concoction 112–113
Cherryfields Clinic 112
chi 49, 84, 101, 103, 108, 113
'chicko' oil 75
chrysarobin 40
climatotherapy 64, 69–75
clinical ecology 67–69
coal tar 12, 39–40, 42, 44, 63
cognitive therapy 90
collagen 5, 41
conception 13, 45
conventional medicine 37–46, 47, 48, 52, 55, 56, 60, 62, 69, 76, 77, 97, 99, 109
corticosteroids 39, 40–41
Coué, Emile 87
counselling 91
crab apple 94
creative therapies 92
cyclosporin A 38, 45
cytotoxic therapy 44, 68

dairy products 61
Dead Sea 69, 70–74
Dead Sea mud 71, 74
Dead Sea salts 28, 75
dermis 5, 6, 8, 9

detergent 27, 28, 30
detoxification 60, 65, 67
diet 2, 13, 19, 22, 31, 42, 49,
    56–67
digestive system 56, 59
discoid psoriasis, *see* plaque
    psoriasis
dishidrotic eczema 14
dithranol 39, 40, 44
dock 112
doctor fish 74
doctors, *see* conventional
    medicine
Do-In 108
drugs 23, 34, 37, 38, 48, 60
drugs, side-effects of 38, 41,
    44–45, 48

eccrine glands 6
eczema 11, 13, 14, 59, 61, 67,
    103, 113
eicosapentaenoic acid (EPA)
    20, 22, 62
Ein Bokek 73
Ein Gedi 71
elastin 5
elder 111
elimination diet, *see* exclusion
    diet
emollients 27–29, 39
emotions 4, 18, 20, 38, 48–49,
    76–95, 99
endorphins 32, 103
enkephalins 103
epidermis 4, 8, 41
erythrodermic psoriasis 14
essential fatty acids 62
evening primrose oil 62
exclusion diet 59
exercise 32, 65

fabrics 30–31
Farber, Dr Eugene 18, 21

fasting 65
fish oil 58, 62
flexural psoriasis 12
fumaric acid 63

gammalinoleic acid 62
gestalt therapy 90
graphites 101
group support 71, 72, 91–92
guttate psoriasis 12, 22

Hahnemann, Dr Samuel 96
hair follicles 6
healing crisis 53
hepatitis 74
herbal medicine (Chinese)
    58, 96, 103, 113
herbal medicine (Western)
    31, 36, 55, 64, 75, 96, 108
Hippocrates 96
HIV 74
holistic medicine 48, 96–115
homoeopathy 54, 55, 64, 93,
    96–101
hormones 23, 64, 108, 103
hospital treatment 14, 38
hydrocortisone 41
hypnosis, *see* hypnotherapy
hypnotherapy 88–89

ibuprofen 46
immune system 17–18, 45,
    67, 98
iridology 50
itching/scratching 35, 64, 80,
    101

Jin Shen 108

Keratin 4, 13
Keratinocytes 41
ki 49, 101
kinesiology 50

lanolin 27
lavender 28, 92, 93
leucotrienes 20, 62
lifestyle 21–22, 49, 52, 65, 102
light therapy 43–44
liver 18–19, 41, 44, 45, 56, 57, 99, 102, 109
localized pustular psoriasis 13
lungs 102, 103
lymph glands 6

magnesium 70
masked sensitivity 68
medical dowsing 50
meditation 25, 83–86
melanin 5
melanocytes 5
mental health 3, 20, 24
meridians 51, 101–105
methotrexates 38, 44–45
migraine 80, 103
mind-body link 48–49, 76
minerals 58, 62, 68–69, 112
mora therapy 50–51
mother tincture 97
moxibustion 102
mugwort 102
music therapy 92

nail psoriasis 13
'napkin' psoriasis 13
National Health Service 47, 67, 96
naturopathy 57, 58, 59, 64–65
neuropeptides 18
North American flower remedies 95
nutritional therapy 65–67

pendulum 50
petroleum jelly 39
placebo 54, 76–77, 97

plaque psoriasis 11, 22
plaques 1, 11, 29, 30, 40, 94, 111
pollution 21, 57, 65, 66, 67, 68, 69
polyamines 19, 56
pompholyx 14
pores 6
potassium 41
prana 49, 84, 101
pregnancy 15, 23, 42
professional misconduct 89, 121–122
professional organizations 117, 118–120, 125–129
psoralens 43
psoriasis, in babies and children 13, 35–36
psoriasis, causes and triggers of 3, 8, 16–23, 65–67
psoriasis, chronic nature of 2, 54
psoriasis, emotional effects of 4, 80–81
psoriasis, genetic links with 16–17
psoriasis, other people's attitudes to 1, 23, 24, 34, 35, 80, 81
psoriasis, symptoms of 1, 8, 11–15
psoriatic arthritis 14, 46, 69
psychodrama 91
psychotherapy 89–90
pulse 50, 68
PUVA 43, 74

qi, see chi

RAST test 68
red clover 111
reflexology 96, 114–115
relationships 34

relaxation 18, 25–26, 36, 70–72, 82, 92–93
retinoids 38, 45
rotation diet 66

sandalwood 93
sarsaparilla 111
scaling, see plaques
scalp 12, 30, 42
sebaceous glands 6
sepia 101
serotonin 103
shampoo 29, 30, 42
Shen Tao 108
Shiatsu 108
skin 3, 4–8, 26, 78
skin cells 1, 8, 11, 56, 79
skull-cap 112
sleep 36
smoking 34, 58, 112
spinifex 94
spirulina 64
steroids 23, 39, 40, 73, 74, 99, 100, 105, 108
streptococcus, see throat infections
stress 20, 23, 25–26, 47, 65, 79–80
stress-busters 25–26
sulphur 101
sunlight 23, 32, 63, 64, 69–70
supplements 62–64, 66, 68
systemic therapies 37, 38, 42, 44–46

T'ai chi 84
T-helper cells 17, 45
thermal springs 74

throat infections 22
tiredness 36
tissue salts 64
topical therapies 37, 39–41, 44
toxins 5, 6, 19, 44, 53, 57, 59, 61, 66, 67, 75, 108, 109, 111
transactional analysis 90–91

ultraviolet rays 32, 39, 43, 44, 70
unguentum cocois 42
UVA 32, 43, 70
UVB 32–33, 39, 44, 70, 72

Vacuflex 115
valerian 112
vanilla leaf 95
Vega 50, 68
vesicular dermatitis 14
visualization 86–87
vitamins 58, 62, 69, 112
vitamin A 58, 64
vitamin B complex 58, 62, 64
vitamin C 60
vitamin D 32, 39, 41, 62, 64

Walsh family 112
washing powders 27
watercress 112
water violet 81, 94
wheatgerm oil 93
willow 81, 94

yin and yang 49, 101
yoga 84

zinc 41, 63